Rehabilitation of Older People

JOIN US ON THE INTERNET VIA WWW, GOPHER, FTP OR EMAIL:

WWW: http://www.thomson.com
GOPHER: gopher.thomson.com
FTP: ftp.thomson.com
EMAIL: findit@kiosk.thomson.com

A service of I(T)P[®]

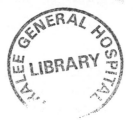

Rehabilitation of Older People

A handbook for the multidisciplinary team

Second edition

Edited by

Amanda J. Squires

Chartered Physiotherapist,
Adviser, Professions Allied to Medicine,
Barking and Havering Health Authority;
Visiting Lecturer, King's College, London and
the UN International Institute of Ageing, Malta.

Consultant editor: Jo Campling

 CHAPMAN & HALL
London · Weinheim · New York · Tokyo · Melbourne · Madras

Published by Chapman & Hall, 2–6 Boundary Row, London SE1 8HN, UK

Chapman & Hall, 2–6 Boundary Row, London SE1 8HN, UK

Chapman & Hall GmbH, Pappelallee 3, 69469 Weinheim, Germany

Chapman & Hall USA, 115 Fifth Avenue, New York NY 10003, USA

Chapman & Hall Japan, ITP-Japan, Kyowa Building, 3F, 2-2-1 Hirakawacho, Chiyoda-ku, Tokyo 102, Japan

Chapman & Hall Australia, 102 Dodds Street, South Melbourne, Victoria 3205, Australia

Chapman & Hall India, R. Seshadri, 32 Second Main Road, CIT East, Madras 600 035, India

Distributed in the USA by Singular Publishing Group Inc., 4284 41st Street, San Diego, California 92105

First edition 1988

Second edition 1996

© 1988 Amanda J. Squires

© 1996 Chapman & Hall

Typeset in 10/12pt Palatino by Mews Photosetting, Beckenham, Kent

Printed in Great Britain by Page Bros. Ltd, Norwich

ISBN 0 412 71930 4   1 56593 735 X (USA)

A catalogue record for this book is available from the British Library

Library of Congress Catalog Card Number: 96-84037

Contents

Contributors

Kirsten Beining BSc(Hons), MRCSLT
Senior Speech and Language Therapist, Western Community Hospital, Southampton, Hampshire

Alison Blenkinsopp PhD, BPharm, MRPharmS
Director of Education and Research, Keele University Department of Pharmacy Policy and Practice, Staffordshire

Chris Drinkwater BA, MB, BChir, DCH, DObstRCOG, FRCGP
Senior Lecturer, Department of Primary Health Care, University of Newcastle upon Tyne, Tyne and Wear; Sir Roy Griffiths Educational Fellow for Older People (an Age Concern/Royal College of General Practitioners/Prince of Wales Fellowship)

Olwen E. Finlay FCSP, HT, DMS
Superintendent Physiotherapist, Department of Health Care for Elderly People, Royal Hospitals, Belfast

Colin J. Fullerton MMedSci, FPodA
Senior Podiatrist, Centre for Podiatric Medicine, The Queens University of Belfast, Belfast

Anne Gale BA(Hons), RGN, RM, RCNT, DN(Lond)
Nurse Teacher, Co-ordinator Rehabilitation Studies, University of Southampton School of Nursing and Midwifery, Faculty of Medicine, Health and Biological Sciences, Hampshire

Jane Gaylard BNSc(Hons), RGN
Quality and Audit Co-ordinator for Elderly Services, Southampton Community Services Trust, Hampshire

James George MB, FRCP
Consultant in Medicine for the Elderly and Director of Rehabilitation, Carlisle Hospitals, Carlisle

Jean Hall MA, DipCOT, SROT
Independent Consultant Occupational Therapist in Private Practice, Jean Hall Associates, Uxbridge, Middlesex

Margaret Hastings BA, MCSP, SRP
Superintendent Physiotherapist, Physiotherapy Services for Older People, Lomond Healthcare NHS Trust, Alexandria

Denise Keir MA, MA(Educ)
Senior Lecturer, Centre for Education Studies, Croydon College, Surrey

Jill Manthorpe MA
Lecturer in Community Care, Department of Social Policy and Professional Studies, The University of Hull, Humberside

Jill Mantle BA, MCSP, DipTP
Senior Lecturer, Department of Health Sciences, University of East London, London

Jane Milligan
Head of Hearing Therapy, Bath and West Community NHS Trust, Avon

Rosemary Oddy MCSP, SRP
Former Head of Leicester Mental Health Physiotherapy Service, Carlton Hayes Hospital, Leicestershire; currently Freelance Advisor in Physiotherapy in Old Age Psychiatry

Janet Pierce DBO(T), Dip Rehab Studies
Orthoptist, Gloucester Royal NHS Trust, Gloucestershire, (Formerly Principal, Chester School of Orthoptics)

Kiran Shukla BSc, BEd, SRD
District Dietician, Thameside Community Healthcare NHS Trust, Essex

Anna Smith MCSP, SRP
Senior Physiotherapist, Bridgend and District NHS Trust, Penarth, Cardiff.

Joyce M. Smith PhD, BDS, MMedSci
Consultant in Dental Public Health, Barking & Havering and Redbridge
& Waltham Forest Health Authorities, London/Essex

Amanda Squires MSc, FCSP, SRP
Adviser, Professions Allied to Medicine, Barking and Havering Health
Authority, Essex

Jane Stephenson BA, MCSP, SRP
Senior Physiotherapist, Berkeley Hospital, Severn NHS Trust,
Gloucestershire

Cameron G. Swift PhD, FRCP
Professor of Health Care of the Elderly, King's College London;
Consultant Physician, King's College Hospital, London

Charles Twining PhD, MA, MSc, AFBPsS
Head of Psychology Services, Cardiff Community Health Care NHS
Trust, Whitchurch Hospital, Cardiff

Fiona Watts BA, MSHAA
Senior Specialist Hearing Therapist, Bath and West Community NHS
Trust, Avon

Jayne Whitaker DipCSLT, MRCLST
Principle Speech-Language Therapist, Southampton University Hospital
Trust, Hampshire

John Young MB, MSc, FRCP
Consultant in Medicine for the Elderly, St Lukes Hospital, Bradford

Acknowledgements

All contributors to the first edition whose work stimulated the need for a further edition. Sally Ann Adams, Jane Stephenson and Anna Smith for editorial assistance.

Chapter 1
J. Gaylard, A. Gayle, J. Manthorpe, R. Oddy, and J. Stephenson, for discipline-specific contributions to the historical perspective.

Chapter 8
Madeline Taylor, co-author of the same topic chapter in the 1st edition, whose valuable contribution on occupational therapy has enabled a balanced picture of therapy to be presented in this chapter.

Chapter 10
Anna Motley for contributing 'home from hospital'.

Bernadette Harrington, Audrey Finer, Maureen English and particularly Rita Eady for assistance with processing the contributions.

Preface

Attitudes to rehabilitation of older people, particularly in departments specializing in care of the elderly, have become increasingly positive in recent years. A growing number of professionals see the speciality as a necessary career experience, and this needs encouragement if the professions are to be prepared for the increasing number of older people who will require help from their members.

The purpose of this book is to bring together the skills and experience of experts in several fields of rehabilitation to provide a primer for those needing the knowledge of how to manage the older person in whatever environment or speciality they present. Readers will be able to enhance their own knowledge already gained in a variety of fields, and play an immediate part in the team. The information will also be of value to interested carers, agencies contributing to the widened provision of service to older people, and their purchasers.

The continuing transformation of healthcare delivery world-wide, resulting from changing user and provider expectations and government policies, is altering approaches to and delivery of rehabilitation services. These current and envisaged future changes are addressed by each discipline, using the UK National Health Service as an example.

Currently many of the clinical judgements made by team members are based on 'experience' or 'intuition', seldom available to the student, newly qualified, or recent returner. In addition the multiple facets of management of the older patient can quickly overwhelm and deter the unprepared. The 'team' concept may also be new and links between disciplines and the services each provides can easily confuse the new participant and be a potential minefield.

We hope, in this book, to have clarified some of these issues.

Rehabilitation of older people – past, present and future

1

Amanda J. Squires

Since publication of the first edition of this book, health and social care in the UK, like many such services world-wide, has undergone fundamental changes. To understand the consequence for rehabilitation of older people and to put the revised chapters which follow into perspective, a review of the history, current changes and the possible future will be outlined.

EVOLUTION OF 'GERIATRICS' AS A SPECIALITY

Current practice in rehabilitation of the elderly is inextricably linked with the historical development of geriatric medicine (Squires, 1986). A variety of institutions, and particularly the family, have always supported the poor, sick and disabled through the centuries. The Middle Ages saw the religious institutions offering help to the poor and sick, although the disabled were often associated with evil and witchcraft or seen as subjects for ridicule. In 1601 the Poor Law introduced the idea of each parish caring for its own poor and a poor rate was levied from parishioners – the forerunner of the community charge. The Poor Law was amended in 1834, centralizing relief for the poor. Parishes were grouped together and the number and size of the workhouses increased. Workhouses accommodated paupers, but their purpose was to deter the poor, rather than to provide care. This resulted in large, grim prison-like institutions to deter admission. The sick poor were accommodated in the adjacent infirmary.

With changes in working practices from home-based agricultural and cottage industries to large-scale factories, the Industrial Revolution, which began during the 19th century, changed the nature of poverty and unemployment; it also promoted the need for more worker mobility and decreased the availability of home-based family help.

The mixing of different categories of paupers (disabled, old, mentally ill and non-disabled poor) in institutions was not altogether changed until the end of the 19th century. Some specific separate categories did develop; for instance those who were blind or deaf were treated separately (French, 1994). The health needs of older people, unfortunate enough to have to enter such institutions, were not considered separately from the poor in general, although poor relief was more likely to be given to them in their own homes.

By the 1930s custodial care for sick older people without resources or family was still generally the norm, often in workhouses. Brocklehurst (1975) suggested that it was not until the state took responsibility for the large number of chronic beds in the public hospital system that the health needs of older people were realized. This occurred largely as a result of the need to relocate 'chronic' patients to make way for those with 'acute' injuries being admitted during the Second World War. The transfer of such large numbers of patients from hospitals to the only large institutions available to take them, workhouse infirmaries, resulted firstly in appalling overcrowding, and secondly in their accompaniment by 'hospital' staff. One such junior doctor was Marjorie Warren, and accounts of what she found and subsequently began to change form a priceless social record (Squires, 1986).

Four groups of patients were described as being found on the chronic sick wards: 'the recovered', comprising a few active patients who, due to their social inadequacy, were kept on by hospitals as staff; 'homeless' individuals; the third and biggest group, the long-stay invalids; and the last and smallest group, those considered to be capable of some response to treatment (Adams and McIlwraith, 1963).

At this time a problem-solving approach to disability, and the concepts of progressive patient care and team work, was added to the acute model of care (accurate diagnosis, classification, prognosis, treatment, cure and discharge). 'Geriatric medicine' as a speciality was born, but has continued to struggle for both recognition and resources in competition with long-established and/or media-attractive specialities.

1948 saw the implementation of the National Health Service (NHS) which was established to meet the medical needs of ill and disabled people as well as providing aids and equipment. The 1947 National Assistance Act provided financial and (Part iii in England and Wales, Part iv in Scotland) residential support for disabled people, under local authority control.

Under the NHS, rehabilitation departments developed to meet the needs of both war veterans and sufferers from the polio epidemic of the early 1950s. Both these events saw a great increase in the number of young disabled people. Rehabilitation replaced convalescence as a means of recovery and instituted the concept of active treatment involving the patient. The 1950s also saw expansion in all industries, including healthcare, and the need to recruit labour from outside the UK – particularly countries with previous colonial connections.

The structure of the rehabilitation team comprised a core group of healthcare professionals – doctors, nurses, physiotherapists and occupational therapists, possibly with some untrained or volunteer support workers. Social work input continued to form a link between hospital and community support services (Chapter 12), but did not develop significantly until the 1970s.

Thus the process of rehabilitation was one of 'hands on' work by professionals, and although 'active', this was in terms of activity decided by the team and for the patient to carry out. The process of rehabilitation looked at restoring optimum function following impairment due to illness or injury and took place over many weeks, months or even years within the one setting. Equipment used was generally an adaptation of traditional gymnastic apparatus. Traditionally, the rehabilitation team has been medically led and in many cases this still applies, but in many locations this is changing, with the professional most appropriate to the case taking the lead and associated responsibility.

SUPPLY AND DEMAND

The need for large-scale rehabilitation provision for older people is relatively recent, for a number of reasons, including the following.

- High infant mortality meant that fewer had survived childhood.
- Short life expectancy (48–50 years in 1900, 55–60 years in the 1940s) meant that few had survived into old age.

General changes in society have also influenced the need for healthcare as well as other services. These are often considered under the acronym STEP, for which a few illustrative examples are provided.

SOCIAL

- Women have achieved greater emancipation and are increasingly part of the paid labour force.
- The nuclear family has replaced the extended family to a large extent.

TECHNOLOGICAL

- Sanitation and nutrition have dramatically increased survival.
- Medical technology has increased opportunities for survival at all ages – the need for the large 'Victorian' family as insurance against low infant survival has decreased.
- Mass immunization programmes and public health measures have increased survival.
- Information technology has enabled the fast transmission of vast amounts of data, enabling the availability of new treatments to be widely known.

- Technology can facilitate independence for people with disabilities.
- Disabling environments can be challenged.

ECONOMIC

- Value for money is stressed by an increasingly discriminating population.
- Concern over public expenditure still dominates political debate.

POLITICAL

Toffler (1981) has indicated:

- a move to the 'right' with increasing affluence and decreasing manual work;
- a decrease in altruism.

Demographers consider a population to be aged if 7% of its number are 65 years or older (Hendricks and Hendricks, 1977). At present in the UK there are approximately 9 million people who are over the age of 65, and by 2021 this is likely to increase to 11 million (Tinker *et al.*, 1994) both exceeding the 7% criterion. However, it is the steadily continuing growth in the numbers of those aged 85 years or over which is changing the distribution of age in the population; in 1991 there were 751 000 and by 2011 it is expected that there will be 201 000 people aged 85 or more in the UK (Coni, Davidson and Webster, 1984).

The combination of these various factors has led to changes in supply and demand for a number of services, including health and social care. These include factors such as the following.

- The need for healthcare increases with age (people over 65 use half the NHS resources).
- The health needs of older people are less acute and more functional.
- Capital resources are redirected to provide more cost-effective care in people's own homes.
- There are fewer adults available for full-time informal or paid care.
- Expectations of all products and services are increasing (we all expect and complain more).

REFORM OF HEALTHCARE

To respond to all these demands the NHS as well as similar systems world-wide has undergone major reform. Although there had been 'tinkering' with the system since 1948, by 1990 it was still a fundamentally mid-20th century system trying to cope with 21st century expectations. The reforms, which are well described in detail elsewhere (Department of

Health, 1989), are based on the purchaser/provider market principle. Health authorities hold the total budget responsibility for their defined population, but hand over agreed proportions as general practitioners (GPs) meet the requirements to become 'fund holders'. Following an assessment of the needs of the population, services are specified, purchased and monitored. The principal issues are as follows.

ASSESSMENT OF NEED

The needs, rather than historical demands, of the population must be assessed. This requires demographic, epidemiological and qualitative studies and should help to identify unmet needs of ethnic and other minority populations, whose poor take up (demand) of services has resulted in inequitable provision. The findings, for example an increased incidence of osteoarthritis of the hip and the desire for pain relief, will be considered alongside credible published reports of effective intervention, in this case perhaps hip replacement. Each discipline with contribution to the care plan will be expected to indicate clear criteria, content, duration of episodes and expected outcomes – which are now being sought as evidence for decisions on how best to meet needs.

HEALTH PROMOTION

The need both to reduce the incidence of disease and to encourage a more positive approach by the population to its own health resulted in the publication of the *Health of the Nation* (Department of Health, 1992). This focuses on a small number of specific conditions, in the anticipation that their incidence and prevalence will be reduced, as will therefore the need for healthcare. The problem is that not only are new conditions emerging, AIDS being a prime example, but the current older population is less likely to benefit from such preventive approaches, which in some cases need to be life long for effect.

SPECIFICATION OF SERVICES – QUALITY, COST AND VOLUME

The proven services to meet the identified needs are then specified in terms of quality and volume requirements, along with the resource to be made available. The monopolistic and welfare style of UK healthcare has resulted in an imbalance of power and a traditionally deferent and 'grateful' patient. To stimulate the quality debate from the potentially powerful user perspective, the Government published *The Patient's Charter* alongside the reforms (Department of Health, 1991). This identifies specific standards that the user can confidently expect, such as maximum waiting time for appointments.

CLINICAL AUDIT

The Patient's Charter specifies requirements easily recognized by patient, provider and purchaser, but fails to address the more complex issues around 'clinical autonomy'. It was accepted that this may only be reviewed competently and credibly by peers, and so the requirement for clinical audit has also been incorporated into the reforms.

COMPETITIVE TENDERING

The service specifications can be considered by both traditional and other potential providers. The purchaser must be aware of possible compromises in the drive for advantage, such as reducing the length of stay but failing to provide services in the community which would have been provided for as an in-patient. The different values and experiences held by a wider range of potential providers present opportunities as well as risks.

EVALUATION AND REFINEMENT

The role of monitoring the cost, volume and especially quality aspects of contracts will be increasingly important, as competition has risks as well as benefits. Refinements to the whole process are continually made as needs, resources and quality requirements change, and facilitate the drive for continuous improvement.

REFORM OF SOCIAL CARE

Social care has also been reformed in conjunction with the reform of healthcare to meet the apparent capital and social advantage of increasing home-based care. Social care reform is also a delayed response to social concerns about the effects of institutionalization on both patients and staff, revealed in damning reports (Martin, 1984).

COMMUNITY CARE

To facilitate cost-effective healthcare, improved arrangements for care in the community were implemented as part of the NHS reforms and have been well described by Neuberger and Sutcliffe (1995). Those for whom discharge is being planned and who are felt to need ongoing care, as well as those already in the community, can be assessed for their needs. This procedure is the responsibility of local authority social services departments, but other members of the health and social team may need to be involved, to ensure that a comprehensive picture is drawn.

The result of the assessment is a 'statement of need', developed with and agreed by the user and their carer. The ensuing care plan can be implemented by care managers, using their allocated budgets, and making use of local, perhaps non-traditional, services. Again, this may reveal a range of differing values that will need to be considered. The individual, family, friends and carers are now considered as major contributors to the rehabilitation process and are expected to take more responsibility for the rehabilitation programme and its outcome and in return expect to be consulted. Access to appropriate health or social respite care will be essential to retain the goodwill of informal carers shouldering the responsibility of community care.

Where care at home is not possible, referral can be made for residential or nursing home care. This may attract financial support from local authorities or may be paid for by the individual out of income and capital.

WORKING IN THE COMMUNITY

Professionals from both health and social services whose work is included in the user's care plan will need to plan their appropriate intervention and regularly review progress. Where the resulting care is of a routine nature and not needing the time of the professional for the intervention, support workers can make a cost-effective contribution, trained and supervised by the professional on a regular basis.

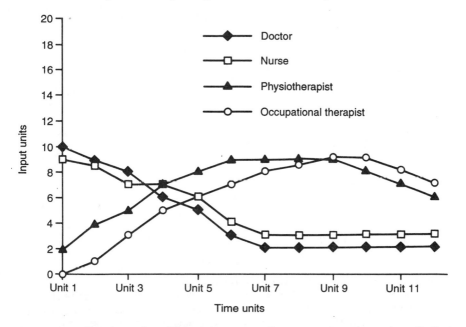

Figure 1.1 The input by different team members over time for a hypothetical rehabilitation patient. Typically there is intensive medical and nursing input on admission, exchanged for therapists' input as time goes on.

Staff working in the community can feel very isolated. Those who lack experience are likely to feel particularly vulnerable. They may be faced with some very threatening problems and need the support of a well organized and understanding management structure. Professional workers who are the sole representative of their profession on the team should have access to a senior colleague for support and advice. Membership of formal 'special interest groups' enables those who work in the same profession and speciality to meet each other for educational and support purposes, the exchange of information and ideas, and the development of research.

If the rehabilitation process is begun in the hospital setting it now lasts for a much shorter period of time and rarely covers the completed episode. Often the process of rehabilitation has barely started at discharge. Squires' (1995a) service input profile (Figures 1.1 and 1.2) shows the empirical level of each professional's input during a hypothetical patient career.

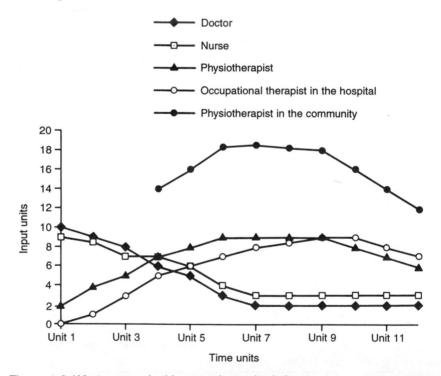

Figure 1.2 What occurs, in this example to physiotherapy, when the hypothetical patient is discharged – often just at the time of increasing therapy need? The time constraints of travel and the social requirements of being a visitor in the patient's home mean that in effect the therapy input is at least doubled for the same patient, but in a different venue. When this factor is multiplied by the number of disciplines affected, the need to cost a complete episode of care becomes apparent, as does the need to share skills appropriately.

Contributing to the doubling of input units are the challenges of rehabilitation in the community setting in terms of time spent travelling, communicating and observing the social requirements of visiting the patient's own home. For instance, the patient and/or carer will feel more confident in discussing problems and asking questions in their own environment. On the hospital ward they often perceive themselves as taking up the professional's valuable time or the professionals appear unable to give them the time for discussion.

A survey in 1992 carried out amongst physiotherapists who were working with older people in the community showed that almost one-third of their time was spent in travelling and communicating with other members of the multidisciplinary team (ACPSIEP, 1993). Contracting arrangements should include such time that is patient-based, but not based on patient contact. Communicating between team members in whatever setting is extremely important, whether between themselves or with the user and their carer. There should be shared goals agreed and set with the team and user, and regular reviews made to measure change. In the hospital setting this can take the form of the weekly ward round, which brings the team together. In the community setting this can be more challenging; there may be a venue for regular meetings, for example at the health centre, or it may be that members of the team can also meet more appropriately at the individual's home. Much of the work of communicating has to take place over the telephone or via the written word. This is time consuming, can make the process of rehabilitation longer and is reliant on adequate documentation.

Poor communication can lead to frustration on all sides which results in a fragmented service with many individual programmes of treatment being carried out that do not have shared goals. This is very confusing, not only for the recipient and carer but also for the professionals involved.

THE FUTURE

There can be no doubt about the continuing drive for cost-effective quality health and social care. This will result in decreasing hospital-based care to 'hub and spoke' centres of excellence. Additional revenue may be needed to meet the costs entailed through reduced caseload capability. The assessor of, and provider of, care may be different, and although the former is necessarily a trained professional, the latter may not need to be. In addition technology has the capability to replace some human tasks. The role of the professional as a teacher or treater of those in need requires consideration by both providers and purchasers.

The delivery of care will be demanded in a style more convenient to the recipient than to the provider. Time of day and goal of the intervention will be more 'user led'. Information on the various services will be sought and compared by purchasers and potential users. The former will seek evidence, the latter softer quality measures as proxy for competence. As part of this drive for contracts of care, users will be expected to play their part. Non-compliance with a programme, non-attendance at an appointment and so on, may be grounds for discharge from the programme. Users' satisfaction with the care provided, measured through various forms of intelligence such as surveys, complaints, take up and outcomes, should be used to support future commissioning decisions.

Professional providers will also undergo change. The 'job for life' expectation has ended, and so a range of skills will need to be developed to meet innovative requirements for time-limited and part-time contracts. Training of all staff, both professionals and others, will require revision to keep pace with the times. Squires (1995b) gives a wider view of the possible future direction of care.

Rehabilitation will take place within many settings for user convenience, not just the specialist centre. Examples include hospitals (acute and community), day hospitals, out-patient centres, health centres, GPs' surgeries, people's own homes, residential and nursing homes.

What is apparent is that care of older people requires different attitudes based on a wide range of skills.

SUMMARY

To meet the health- and social care challenges for all stakeholders in the rehabilitation of older people, the following seem prudent.

- An appreciation of change, market principles and commissioning (Chapter 1);
- An appreciation of demographic, epidemiological and qualitative need (Chapter 2);
- The different needs of minority groups (Chapter 3);
- Consideration of the different values held by stakeholders (Chapter 4);
- Psychological approaches (Chapter 5);
- The skills for successful team working (Chapter 6);
- Effective assessment as the prelude to successful care (Chapter 7);
- An understanding of the perspectives and skills of different disciplines (Chapters 8–16), including:
     proven effectiveness
     outcome measures
     skill mix and delegation
     quality standards;
- An overview and vision of the future of rehabilitation with older people (Chapter 17).

The ensuing chapters should meet at least some of these needs.

REFERENCES

ACPSIEP (1993) *Physiotherapy Staffing Levels for Older People: ACPSIEP Recommendations*, Chartered Society of Physiotherapy, London.

Adams, G.F. and McIlwraith, P.L. (1963) *Geriatric Nursing: A Study of the Work of Geriatric Ward Staff*, Oxford University Press, London.

Brocklehurst, J.C. (ed)(1975) *Geriatric Care in Advanced Societies*, MTP, Lancaster.

Coni, N., Davidson, W.I. and Webster, S. (1984) *Ageing: the Facts*, Oxford University Press, Oxford.

Department of Health (1989) *Working for Patients. The Health Service: Caring for the 1990's*, HMSO, London.

Department of Health (1991) *The Patient's Charter: Raising the Standard*, HMSO, London.

Department of Health (1992) *The Health of the Nation. A Strategy for Health in England*, HMSO, London.

French, S. (1994) In whose service? A review of the development of services for disabled people in Great Britain. *Physiotherapy*, **89**(4), 200–4.

Hendricks, J. and Hendricks, C.D. (1977) *Ageing in Mass Society: Myths and Realities*, Winthrop, Cambridge, Massachusetts.

Martin, J.P. (1984) *Hospitals in Trouble*, Blackwell, London.

Neuberger, J. and Sutcliffe, A. (1995) Community care. *British Journal of Health Care Management*, **1**(6), 311–13.

Squires, A. (1986) Evolution of a speciality. *Therapy Weekly*, **12**(31), 5–6.

Squires, A. (1995a) Physiotherapy staffing levels for older people: case study on fractured neck of femur, presentation to *World Confederation of Physical Therapy*, June, Washington, USA.

Squires, A.J. (1995b) Future directions for the role of the physiotherapists in the care and treatment of older people, in *Physiotherapy in the Care and Treatment of Older People* (eds B. Pickles, A. Compton, A.C. Cott *et al.*), Saunders, London.

Tinker, A., McCreadie, C., Wright, F. and Salvage, A.V. (1994) *The Care of Frail Elderly People in the UK*, HMSO, London.

Toffler, A. (1981) *Third Wave*, Pan Books, London.

Disease and disability in older people – prospects for intervention

2

Cameron G. Swift

INTRODUCTION

In spite of much progress, the provision of healthcare for older people is still often perceived as a problem rather than as a stimulating challenge awaiting professional application. Overriding considerations of a rapidly expanding dependent elderly population confronting a fixed system of supply and demand for services have often led to negative and defensive strategies, which stifle innovation and engender professional reluctance towards the old and their particular healthcare needs.

This chapter argues the case against such an approach by tracing the principles that have emerged from the evolution of modern geriatric medicine, together with some of the documented achievements. In this way, appropriate, tangible and positive objectives are identifiable, opening the way to further progress. Without these, the older members of our society, particularly the more vulnerable, are at risk of continued disservice. While resource provision is an obvious and critical factor, the author's personal view is that many problems have their origin in concept rather than quantity, in professional practice rather than in plant. The philosophy underlying this volume is the potential for intervention and treatment as distinct from accommodation and 'care', and it is therefore appropriate to begin with a consideration of objectives.

PRINCIPLES

The emergence of the medicine of old age as a defined discipline has been based on a composite foundation of principles, including the following.

1. 'Normal' ageing may be compatible with good health.
2. Care and skill in the diagnosis and treatment of disease in older people are both appropriate and fundamental to sound management.
3. Assessment of function – physical, mental and social – should always occur in parallel with medical diagnosis and treatment.
4. Difficulties in diagnosis and assessment commonly occur because of atypical disease presentation and concurrent disorder. Access to the full investigational and treatment facilities of mainstream hospitals is therefore essential.
5. Organized professional team work and efficient linkage to other informal and statutory agencies are necessary at all stages.
6. The skills of problem identification and multidisciplinary 'management by objective' are at least as important as those of standard medical diagnostic and treatment regimens.
7. The capacity of older people to recover from illness and regain complete or partial independence should not be underestimated.
8. The organization of care should be so structured as to eliminate delay, minimize personal disruption and ensure continuity of information and professional contact.

HISTORICAL PROGRESS

The extent to which these interdependent concepts have been developed and given organized expression has largely governed the 'success' or otherwise of healthcare services for the elderly in any locality. The cardinal achievement has been the shift in emphasis from custodial care to successful therapeutic intervention – an investment in the capacity of older people to respond to treatment and in the willingness of a caring community network to stay involved in helping them with the practical problems of independent daily living.

DEFINING AND CALCULATING THE NEED

Quantitative measurement of this process has often been somewhat crude, focusing on hospital activity (such as waiting times, number of admissions and discharges and duration of stay) rather than results for patients themselves. There is an ongoing need to refine and standardize clinically orientated measures of therapeutic performance in the care of older people. To some extent this is because 'need' in service terms can only be defined in terms of a range of possible outcomes. Such measures need to be sensitive and specific to the variables presented, and also amenable to documentation by professionals involved in the busy task of day-to-day service provision.

Some standards of service delivery have, nevertheless, been set. These have involved elimination of delay in intervention, access to high-quality care and treatment, and prospects for successful restoration to community living after significant illness. The performance and efficiency of any future initiatives should be assessed with reference to these if the clock is not to be turned back (see Achievements in the delivery of care, below).

A common conflict affecting professionals involved in rehabilitation is between (1) the entirely appropriate drive to develop, refine and document new techniques and interventions; and (2) the equally appropriate pressure to ensure the continuation of a service to individuals in need within finite resource constraints. This should be perceived as an exciting challenge requiring the closest possible co-operation between the research community and those responsible for day-to-day service provision. The current strategy for research and development in the UK NHS has gone some way towards promoting this interaction.

Such standards should also govern the type and amount of resource provision in order to address the challenges posed by demographic trends. The latter are the subject of a number of recent reviews (e.g. Muir-Gray, 1991; Grundy, 1992; Age Concern Institute of Gerontology, 1992; Warnes, 1993). The overall projections for Britain may be summarized as follows.

1. Currently, 20% of the population is over 60, compared with 7.5% at the beginning of the century. By 2021 the proportion is expected to rise to 24.3%.
2. The elderly population is itself ageing. Over the last 25 years the proportion of over 60s who are older than 75 has risen from a quarter to a third. By 2021, those aged over 75 are projected to account for 8% of the total population.

The male : female ratio in old age is broadly about 1 : 3, probably because of the protective effects of oestrogens against atheroma and the hitherto more hazardous lifestyle pursued by men (including the effects of the World Wars, smoking, alcohol, reckless driving and homicide).

In determining service provision, other demographic characteristics, such as the relative numbers of supporting adults, migration patterns of elderly people and their families, changes in family structure, economic status and available of adequate housing all require proper scrutiny. Of particular significance is the traditional role played by women of working age in caring for older relatives. This is likely to change with current patterns of increased employment and careers for women. Migration is another issue of importance. In the UK, for example, large numbers of older people migrate to certain coastal or rural retirement communities, whilst the families of many living in deprived inner city areas have moved away to the suburbs or beyond. It is important to recognize that these factors may influence not only social structure, but also health, and that a corresponding provision of Health Service resources will therefore be required.

The size of the wage-earning work force has generally decreased and the numbers of older people themselves in employment have also fallen. The net effect of this is to give rise to an increase in the 'dependency ratio', a source of major anxiety to political economists. Against this backdrop it is, however, important to recognize the substantial role played by older people themselves as carers. Investment in this major resource will clearly be a prudent focus of health policy, but it is also a key element for day-to-day clinical practice, affecting the professions concerned with rehabilitation.

INTERRELATIONSHIP OF DISEASE AND DISABILITY IN OLDER PEOPLE

It is well known that a number of diseases which cause disability become more common with advancing age, although this is clearly not always the case, as with (for instance) the demyelinating diseases. Examples include cerebrovascular disease, Parkinson's disease, dementia and the commoner forms of arthritis and osteoporosis. In addition, some diseases encountered in older people are often at an advanced stage of progress, for example chronic airflow obstruction or ischaemic heart disease. Other conditions, such as normal pressure hydrocephalus and pseudo-gout are more particularly 'old-age disorders'.

ILLNESS AND FUNCTION

These and a range of other disorders, together with a reduction in physiological and functional 'reserve' resulting from the normal ageing process, constitute the backdrop against which the modern acute and preventive medicine of old age is practised.

The level of function achieved by an older person with one or more such conditions may remain remarkably stable (if suboptimal) for long periods. When, however, an acute intercurrent disease (e.g. infection) or exacerbation of one of the underlying pathologies (e.g. cerebral or myocardial infarction) occurs, the immediate effect on function is often dramatic, so that the whole range of disorders presents in the form of a functional or social crisis, with or without clear-cut signs of the acute disease itself.

Successful management of such complex clinical situations requires an immediate response, skilled assessment and highly organized team work if the risk of long-term dependency is to be avoided. It is very difficult, as a rule, to predict the range and scale of problems from an initial presumptive diagnosis. The likelihood that these will be considerable does, however, increase exponentially with age. This is apparent from cohort population studies, such as the OPCS Disability Survey (Martin, Meltzer and Elliot, 1988), which identifies an approximate doubling of the prevalence of disability with each successive decade over the age of 50 years. Of those aged 70–79, 41% were found to have some level of disability, with 4% in the severest category. In a longitudinal 4-year follow-up study in the United States for changes in mobility status of 6981 men and women aged 65 and over, 36.2% suffered mobility loss. Increasing age and lower income levels were strongly associated with this, even after controlling for the presence of chronic conditions at baseline. Furthermore, the occurrence during the study of a new heart attack, stroke, cancer or hip fracture was associated with a substantially greater risk of mobility loss than was the presence of these conditions at baseline. An important subset of this analysis additionally showed a major concentration of disability during the 3 years prior to death (Guralnik *et al.*, 1991, 1993).

Analysis of UK hospital in-patient data, which characteristically show an exponential increase with age in the predicted duration of stay (particularly over the age of 75), further emphasizes the importance of this perception for both service policy makers and clinicians.

ACHIEVEMENTS IN THE DELIVERY OF CARE

Measuring progress in the health care of the elderly will never be easy. Few indicators of 'success' enjoy universal acceptance, and there is at times heated controversy amongst the general public, health and social services professionals, informal carers, administrators and even older people themselves as to what is desirable. While some of this debate may be useful in focusing attention on the needs of older people, lack of consensus can also be a major barrier to concerted action, and it is important to identify common objectives.

DEVELOPMENTS IN THE UK

Under the umbrella of the NHS, the early lessons of rehabilitation of older people (Chapter 1) were cumulatively applied to a greater or lesser extent across the health districts of the UK, with increasing recognition of the eight principles outlined earlier. The value of specialist departments based in mainstream district general hospitals, offering immediate access for medically ill old people to the full range of diagnostic, assessment, treatment and remedial facilities, and staffed by physicians and professional co-workers with specific accountability for their care, was set out in several published studies (Hodkinson and Jefferys, 1972; Bagnall *et al.*, 1977; Evans, 1983; Rai, Murphy and Pluck, 1985; Horrocks, 1986; Mitchell, Kafetz and Rossiter, 1987).

MEASURING HEALTHCARE PERFORMANCE

As stated above, the reported outcome has commonly been in terms of hospital activity. Total numbers of hospital beds per head of the older population have been dramatically reduced, waiting lists and bed blockage have been abolished, the throughput of patients has been greatly increased (typically 12 or more patients per bed per year, some 10–15% only of beds at any one time being occupied by patients staying in hospital more than 6 months) and overall average duration of stay reduced to 20–30 days. Such departments have been characterized by a clearly defined role in the acute medical care of older patients, by operational policies promoting continuity of care, by efficient liaison with the community and with other hospital services (usually by means of a central information/liaison office) and by positive policies of rehabilitation and discharge, with well developed multidisciplinary team work (Horrocks, 1986).

The contribution to 'community care' made by this hospital orientated model has consisted, to some extent, in its accessibility to, and dialogue with, general practitioners, district nurses, social services staff, informal carers and other community-based agencies. Respite admissions and day hospital activity feature prominently. Other important consequences have included the ready recruitment of high-quality professional staff, the obvious scope for training and research, and clear-cut departmental 'identity'.

Viewed in the historical context, it can be argued that clear benefits for patients have been achieved, notably removal of the problems of access to hospital treatment without delay and of the fear of waiting to 'go into hospital to die'. Relatives and other carers retain an involvement, sustained by organized support and the knowledge that rescue in a crisis or planned relief are available without delay. These are important criteria of progress with which few would disagree. They constitute documented evidence of a workable balance between community and hospital care, based on professional commitment within the framework of a defragmented service. Such a framework is critical, since fragmentation of care is a particular hazard faced by older people if their multiple or recurring problems are addressed solely by the various agencies of a system-specialized medical service, with disjointed community support and no planned co-ordination.

Rehabilitation of older people after illness must also be perceived and evaluated in the context of such a comprehensive service. It may otherwise run the risk of becoming a self-perpetuating activity concerned more with the role of its practitioners than with the service needs of its recipients.

The methodology for measuring outcome shows some evidence of progress, particularly with the advent of a small number of controlled intervention studies using clinical outcome criteria and avoiding confounding factors within the framework of a randomized prospective design (see Measuring outcome below).

DEVELOPMENTS IN EDUCATION

The logical movement of specialist departments into mainstream hospitals has provided the foundation for medical education in the care of older people. Organized teaching of undergraduate medical students in this discipline now takes place in all UK medical schools and, to a varying extent, in many medical schools in the United States, Canada, Australasia and Europe. Academic departments of geriatric medicine or healthcare of the elderly have expanded, providing a focus for research into the medicine of old age, the processes of ageing and the delivery of care. The involvement of a wide range of professions, including nurses, therapists and social workers, in the formal education of medical students and staff is increasingly promoted in most modern departments. Specific training in the special needs of older people is represented to a varying degree in the curricula of these professions themselves.

COMMUNITY CARE

Much of the above discussion has centred on the historical development of hospital-based services. It is well known, however, that the care of the elderly is undertaken predominantly outside hospitals or institutions, although the hospital constitutes a focus of concentrated acute need and high dependency. Since most older people are likely to experience some hospital contact at some stage, the role of hospital care and its relationship to the community is a major determinant of the long-term outcome they obtain. Prospects for community living, particularly if there is a disability, depend fundamentally on the range of accommodation and services available. These services include primary medical care, community nursing and health visiting, remedial therapy, clinical psychology, chiropody, dental, ophthalmic and audiological services, social work, residential care, home care and day care (Horrocks, 1986). They also depend on a strong partnership between hospital and community care and between health and social services. There is justifiable concern about the outcome of some recent healthcare policies that have strengthened the distinction, and to some extent division, between these key agencies (Department of Health, 1989). While in theory providing a basis to identify the needs of a greatly under-resourced community care sector, the concept of 'substitution' of one for the other is almost certainly fallacious, and may be prompted by the wish to reduce the overall costs of hospital care. In reality, the truly cost-effective goal is to ensure the free flow of older people across the divide between sectors as determined by clinical and personal need. Service strategies based on demarcation or substitution are more likely to result in the recrudescence, demographically driven growth and escalating cost of a continuing inappropriately high demand for continuing institutional care.

An important point is that older people are often unaware themselves of their entitlement, a problem that the voluntary organization, Age Concern, has sought to address over the years. Housing may be a critical factor, and its poor standard often reflects the low economic status of many older people, especially in large urban areas. Re-housing at a later stage is often declined by very elderly people, so that forward-looking policies are necessary for the future, while a responsive and flexible approach to adaptations is needed now.

Sheltered housing with warden cover is a growth industry, but where such resources are limited there are difficulties in rationalizing their use according to need.

Relatives and informal carers continue to constitute the mainstay of community and long-term care. The importance of the enabling role of health and social services by providing adequate support, advice and relief has already been mentioned and cannot be over-stressed. Rejection by relatives is the exception rather than the rule, and is usually the result of too little support too late. Voluntary bodies, including Age Concern and the Association of Carers, have done much to highlight the importance of their critical contribution and their needs are also receiving greater recognition in research (e.g. Homer and Gilleard, 1990, 1994; Williams and Fitton, 1991; Jones and Peters, 1992; Jones and Lester, 1994).

Effective liaison between social services and health service provision is vital for several reasons, but particularly to ensure that scarce community resources are used economically to meet genuine need and that health problems presenting as social crises do not go unrecognized and untreated. The hospital-based social worker, as a member of the multidisciplinary team for healthcare of the elderly, has historically played a vital role in this respect, not only in case work with older people and their carers, but also in providing the operational link with residential care, home helps, meals services, day centres, voluntary agencies, housing departments and community care schemes. Recent policies promoting an erosion of this role can only hinder progress or prove detrimental.

The critical challenge ahead is to eliminate fragmentation of care in the community as well as in the hospital. The activities of any one discipline, whether it be medicine, nursing, remedial therapy, social work or voluntary agency, may at best be wasted or at worst be harmful, if they are not related to an agreed assessment and planned programme of care involving an integrated team.

PROSPECTS FOR THE FUTURE

MEASURING OUTCOME

The medicine of old age incorporates a shift in emphasis from the reduction of mortality to the prevention of morbidity, a goal which is much more difficult to quantify.

A common error is to deduce the type and quantity of service provision required from single time-point prevalence studies. The assumption is made, for example, that the amount of perceived disability in a community at any one point in time indicates the need for 'support' and 'accommodation', when in fact the need may be for better and earlier intervention. Such an approach fails to recognize that health problems in old age and their functional and social consequences commonly follow an acute, rapidly changing, recovering and relapsing pattern, a pattern that may be profoundly affected by the availability or otherwise of skilled diagnosis and properly organized treatment.

What is absolutely clear is the central importance of measuring function as a component of well-being or ill health in older people, an exercise that has been conspicuously neglected by doctors in the past (and to some extent, the present!). Recent studies in stroke (which is in some respects an excellent model for rehabilitation of older patients in general) have highlighted the usefulness of functional prognostic indicators as predictors of medium and longer-term outcome, focusing on their superiority over neuroanatomical and other more conventional diagnostic categories, as well as their applicability to typical populations of older patients (Kalra and Crome, 1993).

In the development of functional assessment scales, physiotherapists have led the way and there is much excellent published work. The subject of functional assessment is explored in detail later in this book. To date, none of the many rating scales and 'quality of life' measures devised has been shown to have optimal sensitivity or specificity, nor have they achieved universal acceptance in any one domain of clinical outcome assessment or cost effectiveness. The necessary experimental studies are often overwhelmed by the drive to achieve quick-fix audit criteria. On the other hand, operational evaluation studies commonly require very large numbers in multiple centres to produce a study of adequate power. Under these circumstances, the selection of outcome criteria may be a compromise based on consensus and pragmatism – without which the study could not be undertaken at all. In research terms, it all depends on the precise question being asked. Ideally, the two approaches – (1) developing sensitive outcome measures; and (2) measuring broad service effectiveness – need to go hand in hand, a balance to be struck by research grant-giving bodies.

A third, but crucial, research method is the smaller or intermediate scale controlled intervention study. This is analogous to a phase 2 or 3 clinical trial in drug development, characterized by a tightly defined study population sample, a degree of standardization of both the intervention and the measures of outcome and a prospective random-ized protocol with some element of blinding. These studies are difficult to mount, but are often the only way to reach anything approaching a firm conclusion about a form of treatment. They are gradually beginning to permeate a health service research literature historically peppered with descriptive data, confounding variables and inferences unsup-ported by hard evidence.

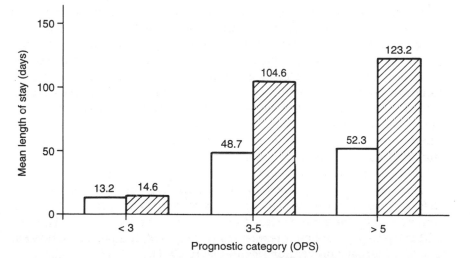

Figure 2.1 The effect of treatment setting (stroke rehabilitation unit, white bars, v. geriatric medical wards, hatched bars) on duration of in-patient stay in a prospective randomized controlled comparative study. The difference between control and intervention groups was significant for those stratified into intermediate (3–5) and poor (> 5) prognostic categories using a validated scale (the Orpington Prognostic Scale). Data of Kalra, Dale and Crome (1993).

Figure 2.1 shows some data from such a controlled study of stroke rehabilitation in a specialized unit compared with existing rehabilitation practice dispersed across more general wards. In this randomized, prospective evaluation, the patient populations were unselected, but stratified into three prognostic categories, the patient characteristics and therapy interventions were clearly documented and comparable between control and intervention groups, and the results showed the benefit of tightly focused multidisciplinary practice (i.e. the stroke unit) on a number of key indicators of clinical and service outcome. Had a retrospective comparison been undertaken, say between two different centres, no firm conclusion could have been drawn, because of the possibility of a whole range of confounding variables. There is an urgent need for more experimental work of this kind.

PREVENTION

So far we have concentrated on how health problems are managed and treated when they present, typically as some form of acute crisis or breakdown in function, and have emphasized that the skilfulness or otherwise of such management may profoundly influence the subsequent prospects for independent living of older people and the numbers requiring long-term institutional care. In other words, good treatment of illness in old age has, to some extent, a preventive function.

A common reaction, however, is to say 'if only this particular problem had been dealt with earlier, it might have been much less serious or prevented altogether, irreversible damage might have been averted'. **Primary** prevention in the sense of dealing with the known cause of the condition and so completely preventing its occurrence has been largely, hitherto, an exercise for the medicine of earlier life. Examples would include the common immunizations, elimination of asbestos exposure and perhaps the elimination of tobacco consumption. **Secondary** prevention is concerned with the early detection of disease or its precursors in patients who are asymptomatic and consider themselves fit, and constitutes the rationale for screening programmes.

This can be distinguished from case finding, in which established disease and its consequences are present but for a variety of reasons unreported by the sufferer. Case finding, with a view to earlier diagnosis and the prospect for better results from treatment, has been described as a form of tertiary prevention (Williamson, 1981).

The concept of universal screening of the older population (defined by a given chronological age) has met with little favour, not least because of the unrealistic time required of professional staff (whether general practitioners or other professional health visitors) and the apparently low returns achieved in such a blanket approach. Attention has to some extent been focused more on attempting to define categories of older people who are arguably at risk of health problems and to target case-finding initiatives at these groups, as in an early survey conducted in Aberdeen (Age Concern Research Unit, 1983). This, expanding an earlier World Health Organization (WHO) list, selected the very old (> 80), socially isolated (not necessarily living alone), those without children, those in poor economic circumstances, those recently discharged from hospital, those who had recently changed their dwelling, the divorced/separated and those in social class V (Registrar General's classification). Interestingly, many of these 'conventional' risk factors proved rather inefficient as markers for case finding. An alternative two-stage approach, based on an initial postal screening questionnaire, followed, where appropriate, by a comprehensive health visitor assessment, was also described (Age Concern Research Unit, 1983). This proved somewhat more efficient, and the analysis of findings suggested further economies based on selecting the most discriminating questions identified. The main benefits overall consisted of determining and addressing a number of unmet needs (mainly contact with available services and treatment of active health symptoms). These benefits were clearly demonstrable, and could also be shown to be achievable with feasible changes in doctor, health visitor and district nurse workload.

A number of further studies have been published over the last decade, unfortunately with wide variations in methodology (for example, in the choice of professionals and health assessments employed and in the outcome measures) (e.g. Vetter, Jones and Victor, 1984; Hendriksen, Lund and Stromgard, 1984; McEwan et al., 1990; Carpenter and Demopoulos, 1990; Pathy et al., 1992; Fabacher et al., 1994). An important and positive shift in the thinking underlying screening studies has been towards functional and disability-related outcome criteria rather than medical and pathological outcomes. To date, however, it remains impossible to draw firm conclusions about the possible benefits of screening programmes for older people. A variety of positive outcomes has included a rise in morale amongst those screened, an increase in referrals to all agencies (including specialist medical care), a reduced duration of in-patient stay in some studies and (interestingly) a reduction in mortality. No trial has demonstrated an improvement in functional ability, and the workload of general practitioners appears to be reduced only where alternative services are provided (Iliffe, 1993).

There is an ongoing need for further research. Prevention studies should preferably be undertaken as a joint initiative with viable and well organized hospital-based services whose positive impact in reducing long-term bed occupancy is well attested. There seems little point in embarking on a study of preventive approaches when there is a fundamental deficiency in the ability of services to meet those unmet needs which are so identified. The opportunities for general practitioners, physicians in geriatric medicine and the professionals with whom they work to combine their respective skills in further research with an accent on prevention are clearly most exciting. Some cautionary points, however, emerge from the projects already undertaken, in particular the following.

1. There is a major necessity to refine both markers of need and measures of outcome in the healthcare of older people. This requires careful research and observation, since our current perception of health and ill health determinants, however 'logical', may easily be mistaken.
2. Prevention may well (in time) result in much benefit to many older people, but there is no guarantee that it will make their healthcare cheaper. Indeed, available evidence, in so far as it points up major areas of unmet need, suggests that the opposite may be the case. Therefore, naive planning assumptions about prevention and 'community care' as economical alternatives to current medical practice are seriously ill founded.
3. It follows, therefore, that policy makers and planners should not divert funds wholesale from existing services to new initiatives unless the latter have been thoroughly validated and shown to be of measurable value to the large majority of older people.
4. Resources for well designed controlled prospective intervention studies constitute sound investment (whilst ensuring that existing services that are working well remain adequately supported and are made more uniformly available).

SUMMARY

Disease and disability go hand-in-hand with increasing frequency, the older the sufferer. For many decades, while medical science has advanced technically, the disabilities of the old have met with a passive and negative acceptance by medical practitioners, healthcare providers and many of the population at large. It is now clear, however, that a positive, organized, professional and to some extent specialized approach to diagnosis, assessment and intervention can have a major and positive impact on the prospects for continued autonomy of a large majority of ill older people, and on the burdens carried by relatives, families and caring communities. The collaboration and co-ordination of several professionals and other agencies is a central factor in achieving results. Successful models of healthcare have been developed and described. These require consolidation and wider application. At the same time research into new patterns of intervention with an accent on preventive healthcare is now a clear requirement. It presents a challenge to the commitment and skill of all those concerned to ensure a better future for older people.

REFERENCES

Age Concern Institute of Gerontology (1992) *Life After 60: A Profile of Britain's Older Population*, Age Concern Institute of Gerontology, King's College, London.

Age Concern Research Unit (1983) *Research Perspectives on Ageing, 6; The Elderly at Risk*, Age Concern, London.

Bagnall, W.E., Datta, S.R., Knox, J. and Horrocks, P. (1977) Geriatric medicine in Hull: a comprehensive service. *British Medical Journal*, **2**, 102–4.

Carpenter, G.I. and Demopoulos, G.R. (1990) Screening the elderly in the community: controlled trial of dependency surveillance using a questionnaire administered by volunteers. *British Medical Journal*, **300**, 1253–6.

Department of Health (1989) *Caring for People. Working for Patients*, HMSO, London.

Evans, J.G. (1983) Integration of geriatric with general medical services in Newcastle. *Lancet*, **1**, 1430–3.

Fabacher, D., Josephson, K. *et al.* (1994) An in-home preventive assessment program for independent older adults. *Journal of the American Geriatrics Society*, **42**(6), 630–8.

Grundy, E. (1992) The epidemiology of ageing, in *Textbook of Geriatric Medicine and Gerontology*, 4th edn (eds J.C. Brocklehurst, R. Tallis and H. Fillit), Churchill Livingstone, Edinburgh.

Guralnik, J.M., LaCroix, A.Z., Branch, L.G. *et al.* (1991) Morbidity and disability in older persons in the years prior to death. *American Journal of Public Health*, **81**(4), 443–7.

Guralnik, J.M., LaCroix, A.Z., Abbott, R.D. *et al.* (1993) Maintaining mobility in later life. I. Demographic characteristics and chronic conditions. *American Journal of Epidemiology*, **137**(8), 845–57.

Hendriksen, C., Lund, E. and Stromgard, E. (1984) Consequences of assessment and intervention among elderly people: a three year randomised controlled trial. *British Medical Journal*, **289**, 1522–4.

Hodkinson, H.M. and Jefferys, P.M. (1972) Making hospital geriatrics work. *British Medical Journal*, **4**, 536–9.

Homer, A.C. and Gilleard, C. (1990) Abuse of elderly people by their carers. *British Medical Journal*, **301**, 1359–62.

Homer, A.C. and Gilleard, C. (1994) The effect of inpatient respite care on elderly patients and their carers. *Age and Ageing*, **23**(4), 274–6.

Horrocks, P. (1986) The components of a comprehensive District Health Service for elderly people – a personal view. *Age and Ageing*, **15**, 321–42.

Illiffe, S. (1993) Screening the elderly – two steps forward, one step back?, in *The Medical Annual* (ed J. Fry), John Wright, Bristol.

Jones, D. and Lester, C. (1994) Hospital care and discharge: patients' and carers' opinions. *Age and Ageing*, **23**(2), 91–6.

Jones, D.A. and Peters, T.J. (1992) Caring for elderly dependents: effects on the carers' quality of life. *Age and Ageing*, **21**(6), 421–8.

Kalra, L. and Crome, P. (1993) The role of prognostic scores in targeting stroke rehabilitation in elderly patients. *Journal of the American Geriatrics Society*, **41**, 396.

Kalra, L., Dale, P. and Crome, P. (1993) Improving stroke rehabilitation: a controlled study. *Stroke*, **24**, 1462.

McEwan, R.T., Davison, N., Forster, D.P. *et al.* (1990) Screening elderly people in primary care: a randomised controlled trial. *British Journal of General Practice*, **40**, 94–7.

Martin, J., Meltzer, H. and Elliott, D. (1988) *OPCS Surveys of Disability in Great Britain, Report 1*, HMSO, London.

Mitchell, J., Kafetz, K. and Rossiter, B. (1987) Benefits of effective hospital services for elderly people. *British Medical Journal*, **295**, 980–3.

Muir-Gray, J.A. (1991) Social and community aspects of ageing, in *Principles and Practice of Geriatric Medicine*, 2nd edn (ed. M.S.J. Pathy), Wiley, Chichester.

Pathy, M.S., Bayer, A., Harding, K. and Dibble, A. (1992) Randomised trial of case-finding and surveillance of elderly people at home. *Lancet*, **340**, 890–3.

Rai, G.S., Murphy, P. and Pluck, R.A. (1985) Who should provide hospital care of elderly people? *Lancet*, **1**, 683–5.

Vetter, N.J., Jones, D.A. and Victor, C.R. (1984) Effect of health visitors working with elderly patients in general practice. *British Medical Journal*, **288**, 369–72.

Warnes, A.M. (1993) *The Demography of Ageing in the United Kingdom of Great Britain and Northern Ireland*, International Institute on Ageing, Malta.

Williams, E.I. and Fitton, F. (1991) Survey of carers of elderly patients discharged from hospital. *British Journal of General Practice*, **41**(344), 105–8.

Williamson, J. (1981) Screening, surveillance and case-finding, in *Health Care of the Elderly* (ed. T. Arie), Croom Helm, London.

Rehabilitation and elderly ethnic minorities

3

James George and John Young

INTRODUCTION

The elders of ethnic minorities face a potential triple jeopardy: at risk through old age, through discrimination and through lack of access to health and social services (Norman, 1985). Traditionally, Britain has accepted a variety of ethnic minority groups within its population, so that many different races and cultures are represented in the UK elderly population profile (Table 3.1). In some inner city areas the so-called ethnic minorities are in fact the majority and the number of their elderly is increasing through ageing of the established and the arrival of dependants. In order to provide appropriate care we need to be aware of the background and special health problems and requirements of the ethnic minority groups within the UK population.

Table 3.1 Ethnic composition of the population in England and Wales from the 1991 census

Ethnic group	Number	Percentage of total	Estimate of percentage of pensionable age
White	46 936 500	94.1	19
Black Caribbean	499 000	1.0	5
Black African	205 400	0.4	2
Black other	176 400	0.4	2
Indian	830 600	1.7	4
Pakistani	454 500	0.9	2
Bangladeshi	159 500	0.3	1
Chinese	147 300	0.3	1
Other Asian	193 100	0.4	3
Other	280 900	0.6	5
Total	49 883 200	100	19

DEFINITION

The term ethnic minority group is used to refer to people of any race who see themselves as sharing a common culture which is distinct from that of the majority of the population. Since April 1995 collecting data on ethnic group from all patients admitted to NHS hospitals has been routine and the data are intended to be used to plan appropriate services, assess take up and develop an action plan. Patients are required to indicate their felt ethnicity, which can prove confusing to some older people. The reliability of such data for this age group is a cause for concern.

Health services are required to base their questions on the major census groups – white, black Caribbean, black African, black other, Indian, Pakistani, Bangladeshi, Chinese and other. This may need to be supplemented by adding other locally significant groups – e.g. Vietnamese.

BACKGROUND OF SOME ETHNIC MINORITY GROUPS

Migration of people as individuals or groups has resulted in Britain becoming a multicultural and multi-ethnic society. The reason for migration can be divided into 'push' or 'pull' factors. The pushed group includes refugees from Eastern Europe or, more recently, from Vietnam. Such people may have arrived in Britain in a state of desperation with few possessions, lack of a clear plan for the future, and in poor physical and mental health, speaking only their native language. They may have left important family members behind with no realistic chance of a reunion. They may be bitter and resent the loss of their previous lifestyle. In such cases the migration may be viewed as similar to a 'bereavement' and indeed the person may go through a bereavement-type process including anger, denial, guilt and depression. The situation can be exacerbated by continued political change in their country of origin which may make return impossible and increase the feeling of isolation, with loss of their original links.

In contrast, 'pull' factors operate when an individual or group has been attracted to Britain for self-betterment and a more prosperous way of life. This includes South Asians from the Indian subcontinent and also Afro-Caribbeans shortly after the Second World War. The common pattern is for one member of the family, usually the son, to migrate, often followed by wife and parents. Tensions can arise through the 'resettlement trap' in which the second generation sons and wives stand between two cultures. The first generation have difficulty integrating and generally remain separate in distinct communities, whereas the third generation may become closely integrated into the new 'Western' culture. Thus, competing loyalties may produce tension and conflict.

As in all cultures, comfort is derived from common association, and cultural communities have developed, providing social and retail facilities, making it unnecessary to use mainstream facilities or to learn English. This mirrors the British ex-patriot communities in some Mediterranean countries. The main difference in Britain is that the ethnic minority migrants are generally in the lower socioeconomic groups and have consequently settled in areas of poorer housing stock and other facilities and high unemployment, from which groups ascending the ladder of prosperity have willingly moved on. It is only when reliance is needed on 'majority' facilities – such as emergency health care – that communication problems are exposed.

For minority groups in Britain it should not be assumed that literacy in the native language exists. This is particularly a problem for females in the culture, and other methods of communication should be used. Video use, particularly by Asian elders, probably exceeds that of other elderly groups and can be a useful medium to pursue.

Brief backgrounds of some common ethnic minority groups are now described.

ELDERLY PEOPLE OF POLISH ORIGIN

At the turn of this century many Polish Jews came to the UK, fleeing persecution. The Polish Jews settled mainly in the East End of London, Manchester and Leeds and tended to speak Polish or Yiddish. After the Second World War 100 000 members of the Polish forces stayed in Britain and there were also many wartime refugees. Most of these Poles settled in London, Birmingham, Manchester and Bradford, with smaller populations in Wolverhampton, Leeds, Nottingham, Sheffield, Coventry, Leicester and Slough. The post-war Polish settlers are mostly Roman Catholic, although some are Jews.

ELDERLY PEOPLE OF INDIAN ORIGIN

People came to the UK from two main Indian states: Punjab and Gujarat. The men came in the 1950s and early 1960s and were joined by their families, often many years later. People from the Indian Punjab speak Punjabi and most are Sikh by religion. There are large Punjabi Sikh communities in the West Midlands, Glasgow, West London and Leeds. People of Gujarati origin from India and East Africa live mainly in North and South London, Coventry, Leicester and Manchester. Most are Hindus. Although the national language of India is Hindi, relatively few people of Indian origin speak it as a first language, instead using a regional dialect, though many may speak Hindi as a second language.

ELDERLY PEOPLE OF PAKISTANI ORIGIN

Many people from Pakistan came to Britain during the late 1950s and early 1960s. They came from three main areas – Mirpur in Azad (Free) Kashmir, Punjab Province and North West Frontier Province. As well as their regional language, they will probably speak Urdu. Most people of Pakistani origin live in Yorkshire, Lancashire, Greater Manchester, West Midlands, Cardiff and Glasgow. The majority of Pakistanis are Muslim.

ELDERLY PEOPLE OF BANGLADESHI ORIGIN

Most people from Bangladesh came to the UK in the 1950s and 1960s and settled throughout the country, but especially in the East End of London. Most Indian restaurants are staffed by Bangladeshis. Almost all are Muslim and come from the rural Sylhet district of Bangladesh and speak a Sylheti dialect.

ELDERLY PEOPLE OF VIETNAMESE ORIGIN

Vietnamese refugees are recent migrants. Several thousand Vietnamese now live in Britain and may have come via refugee camps in Hong Kong. The majority came from North Vietnam and most are ethnic Chinese who speak both Cantonese and Vietnamese. Many Vietnamese have become isolated, as placement policies have resulted in many residing in rural areas, far from other Vietnamese families.

ELDERLY PEOPLE OF AFRO-CARIBBEAN ORIGIN

The great majority of elderly people from the then named 'West Indies' came to the UK in the boom period after the Second World War. Many intended originally to return home. Over half the West Indians who came to Britain came from Jamaica; others came from Guyana, Barbados, Trinidad and Tobago. As with other groups, they tend to be concentrated in inner city areas. However, compared to the other groups, they tend to be very stable in terms of domicile, but with a high rate of council house occupation, rather than being owner-occupiers (Barker, 1984). It is important to remember that there are very distinct differences in culture and previous experience between people from different islands in the Caribbean. Many Afro-Caribbeans are Christians; the largest group are Pentecostalists, some are Anglicans or Baptists and a few are Methodists or Roman Catholics. The departure of a 'village protege' to Britain after the War, in the anticipation of prosperous return and marriage, was not often achieved, as a result of the menial occupations that were found on arrival. Consequently, the delay in return has meant that many stayed single and are now lonely and isolated.

RELIGIOUS AND CULTURAL ATTITUDES

To assist rehabilitation staff and service planners, some main points concerning the Muslim, Hindu and Sikh religions are briefly described.

Muslim

Older male Muslim patients may be unaccustomed to dealing with women of professional status. Muslim women may not agree to being examined by a male member of staff and may prefer to have a female chaperone. In adversity, a Muslim is forbidden to despair seeking help through prayers. Ramadan is a month-long period which forms part of the Islamic calendar and is a basic tenet of the Islamic faith. During Ramadam Muslims are required to abstain from food, tobacco and liquids (including water) between the hours of dawn and sunset. However, those who are ill and/or elderly are usually excused.

Hindu

Hinduism is the religion of 80% of the people in India. It involves a strong sense of personal responsibility and the concept that actions and thoughts in the present life determine the circumstances of the next. Hence, illness may engender feelings of passivity and acceptance.

Sikh

The Sikh religion stresses an individual personal relationship with God and involves helping and serving others. All Sikhs should wear the five signs of Sikhism – kesh (uncut hair); kangha (the comb); kara (the steel bangle); kirpan (a short sword); and kaccha (white shorts). The turban is also a visible symbol for Sikh men and has the same importance as the five 'k's. The religious significance of these symbols needs to be appreciated by doctors, nurses and therapists. Religious symbols worn by patients should be afforded the same respect as the Western wedding ring and not be unnecessarily removed (Karseras, 1991).

HOUSING AND SOCIAL ASPECTS OF ETHNIC MINORITIES

Most of the ethnic minority elders are concentrated in the centres of cities where environmental problems are most acute. Asian and Afro-Caribbean households are more likely to live in older housing and to suffer overcrowding (Barker, 1984). Over one-third of Afro-Caribbean elders live alone; 30% of elderly Asians live alone or with a spouse (Karseras, 1991).

Ethnic minority elders still tend to have backgrounds concentrated in unskilled and semi-skilled occupations where they have been more vulnerable to unemployment. Consequently, ethnic minority elderly may tend to rely on minimum state pensions and may live close to the poverty line. Furthermore, language difficulties may make it difficult for ethnic minority elders to receive the appropriate social and housing benefits. It is tempting to assume that support by the close-knit family network of ethnic minorities can in some way compensate for these disadvantages. Unfortunately, this does not seem to be so and the pattern of elderly parents living with their children appears to be changing (Blakemore, 1983). There seems to be a need for more sheltered housing (Age Concern, 1984) and more day centres for ethnic minority groups (Norman, 1985). The booklet *Which Benefit?* (Benefit Agency, 1995) is available in Urdu, Gujarati, Hindi, Punjabi, Bengali and Chinese, as well as English, and should be available in all departments treating elderly ethnic minority patients.

MEDICAL ASPECTS

There has been comparatively little research on the particular medical problems of elderly ethnic minority patients. Asian patients are known to be more likely to suffer from ischaemic heart disease and there may be more delay in their being transferred to coronary care units from casualty departments, presumably because of language difficulties (Lawrence and Littler, 1985). In one London hospital casualty department it was found that 69 (12%) of all patients seen in one week did not have a good command of English (Dawson, Hildrey and Floyer, 1983). Only 19 (28%) of these patients attended with an outside interpreter, usually a friend or relative. Often these outside 'interpreters' were little better than the patients in their command of English.

Use of the *Red Cross Multilingual Phrase Book* (British Red Cross, 1988) can assist in such emergencies. The patient is asked to recognize their written language from a sample list, which even the illiterate can often manage. Relevant questions can then be selected in the appropriate language for which English translations are available. Alternatively, an interpreter for the relevant language can be sought once the language has been identified, and many systems exist, including three-way telephone, enabling almost immediate link up between patient, staff and an appropriate interpreter anywhere in the country.

Hypertension is more frequent in black Africans and Afro-Caribbeans than in the indigenous or Asian groups – a trend that is also seen in the USA (Beevers and Beevers, 1993). These differences in blood pressure partially explain the high incidence of strokes and renal failure in black people, but not why coronary artery disease is relatively uncommon.

In both Afro-Caribbean and Asian populations non-insulin dependent diabetes is more common than in the indigenous population (Burden, 1993). Complications of diabetes are also more common and these include renal damage, cataracts and ischaemic heart disease, but not foot ulcers. The lack of foot problems in Asian diabetics may be due to regular and ritual foot washing, but Sikhs, interestingly, have been found to have problems with lateral foot ulceration, possibly due to sitting cross-legged (Burden, 1993).

Donaldson (1986) surveyed 726 Asians aged over 65 in Leicester. He found that over half the Asian elderly over-75s were not independent in activities of daily living and one-fifth had some urinary incontinence. These findings, however, do not differ greatly from those for the non-Asian population. One major difference was that more Asians over-75s were able to bathe independently than non-Asian elderly (82% compared to 62%). Perhaps this is because of different methods of bathing, as many Asians prefer to shower rather than to sit in a bath. Donaldson also found that only 37% of Asian elderly men and 2% of Asian elderly women were able to speak English. A handful (4%) of Asian elderly were living alone compared to 46% of non-Asians. Only half of the Asians interviewed were familiar with meals-on-wheels or home helps, and very few were receiving any social service help. Nearly 90% were not aware of the chiropody service and only 3% were receiving chiropody help. There is, therefore, considerable lack of awareness of mainstream health care services by minority patients. This leads many to traditional healers and folk remedies which are accessible and acceptable. There is as little evidence of the effects of traditional medicine as there is of some frequently used Western medicine, and an open mind may prove beneficial.

GENERAL APPROACH TO ETHNIC MINORITY PATIENTS IN HOSPITAL

Irrespective of cultural background, illness brings anxiety and distress for the individual and family. Nevertheless, for some ethnic minority patients admitted to hospital, unfamiliarity with the system and separation from their family home and culture can exaggerate the upset involved with illness. This can be magnified by staff who have insufficient knowledge to modify their approach to suit the differing needs of these patients. The cultural differences described apply equally to patients and to staff, and conflicts within the team may occur over plans for treatment, whatever the culture of the recipient, and will need to be handled sensitively.

Hindu, Muslim and Sikh women are embarrassed at having to expose areas of their body. Legs and upper arms should remain covered at all times. Consequently, hospital 'split-back night gowns' may be especially humiliating. Modesty should be maintained as far as possible during nursing procedures and physiotherapy or occupational therapy treatment sessions, especially in open treatment areas. Healthcare services do not always take into account the high value many people place on personal modesty.

Careful explanation, if necessary through an interpreter, tact and negotiation of the most appropriate and acceptable method of performing a task should be the aim. This also fosters a spirit of understanding and concern, which helps minimize feelings of isolation or distress engendered by the hospital admission. This is particularly valuable if the patient has a disabling condition, as the framework will be laid for the necessary close co-operation (often for a long period) between staff and patient. Irritation, impatience and intolerance will be counterproductive and ultimately undermine the rehabilitation process. It should be borne in mind that the feelings of modesty are deeply ingrained and cannot be easily overcome by simple willpower. Empathy and understanding are required.

Similar respect should be paid to religious needs, jewellery, diet and hygiene requirements. Asian patients may prefer to wash in free-flowing water rather than sit in a bath. After using the lavatory, people from the Indian subcontinent usually wash themselves using the left hand. Lavatory paper is not traditionally used in the Indian subcontinent and may be regarded with distaste. Because the left hand is used to wash the private parts of the body, the right hand is normally used for eating and other tasks. Thus, when fixing an intravenous infusion or placing food where the patient can reach it, the right hand should be kept free if possible. Objects should be handed to a patient so that the right hand can be used. The consequences for a patient having a stroke affecting either upper limb will be obvious.

Restrictions on what may be eaten by Muslims are clearly laid down in the Holy Koran and are regarded as a direct command of God. Elderly Muslim patients in hospital will probably need help in working out which foods on the menu are acceptable. Most will stick to a vegetarian diet, since the meat provided is not halal, which means killed according to Islamic Law. Muslims should not eat pork or anything made from pork or pork products, such as sausages, bacon and ham. Alcohol in all forms is forbidden in the Koran, and the composition of medication should be checked and may not be taken by the patient if they are suspicious of the content (see Chapter 15).

Hospitals in many developing countries expect the family to undertake much of the basic care. Illness is shared and generally one family member will always be present at the bedside. The British practice of restricted hospital visiting may need to be relaxed and this would benefit all relatives. It is essential to use the correct name for patients, including the personal name (e.g. 'Mr Rajinder Singh', not just 'Mr Singh'), and this will also aid record keeping when a large section of the population shares a small number of family names.

Attitudes to ill health also differ. Illness is sometimes regarded as something to be suffered, and it is the expected behaviour to remain 'ill' and in bed until full recovery has occurred. Thus, illnesses in which full recovery may not occur without effort (e.g. stroke, arthritis) may need particularly careful management. The concept of active rehabilitation may, therefore, be unfamiliar to many elderly ethnic minority patients.

Sometimes there may be conflict in the family between the elders with traditional views and the children who have become 'Westernized' and may expect the state to provide much of the care. Occasionally, residential care may be regarded with suspicion and arrangements should be made for a visit to a residential home before deciding whether this is an option. The issue of combination/segregation in such homes is complex and many factors may need to be considered, not least of which is food and religious requirements, but also the rich social gain from ethnic mix.

COMMUNICATION ACROSS A LANGUAGE BARRIER

Rehabilitation is a highly active process in which the onus of responsibility of recovery is transferred from the rehabilitation staff to the individual and the carer. It involves the patient re-learning old tasks or making adjustments to allow a new way of life. Two items are essential. Firstly, the patient and family should gain an understanding of the disabling condition and its consequences. This is essentially an education process. Secondly, the patient and family will need to be actively involved in a set of often complex and progressive manoeuvres to maximize recovery of the damaged body system. Adequate communication is the key to success for both these tasks. Many elderly ethnic minority patients, particularly Asians and East Europeans, will have lived in enclaves of their own cultures. Their knowledge of English will consequently be non-existent or rudimentary. Potentially, this produces a major barrier to successful rehabilitation and represents an important initial task for the staff planning rehabilitation programmes.

There are several practical ways in which rehabilitation staff can improve communication with people who speak little or no English and may also be illiterate in their own language. Ideally, it should be possible to use a qualified interpreter who has had training and is skilled in the nuances of the technique. Every hospital should have a list of locally available interpreters. A good interpreter is more than just a translator. He/she must form a relationship with the patient and provide a bridge between two cultures and two sets of expectations. If a qualified interpreter is not available, relatives and friends may be able to help. This has the advantage that the family become closely involved with the rehabilitation programme and are in a better position to maintain recovery following discharge from hospital. However, a degree of care is needed, as sensitive problems sometimes will be encountered, details of which the patient will be reluctant, or unwilling, to communicate through someone he or she knows. If no interpreter is available, it is important that staff take a little more time to check that instructions are understood, observing the points listed in Table 3.2.

Table 3.2 Ways to improve communication

Use a qualified interpreter if possible.

Simplify your English.

Speak slowly and be patient.

Give non-verbal reassurance.

Get the patient's name right and pronounce it correctly.

Keep comprehensive records to avoid repetition.

Check back – check instructions by asking the patient to explain back to you what he/she is going to do.

Try and avoid questions in which the correct answer is simply 'Yes'.

Avoid idioms (e.g. 'spend a penny').

Write down important points on a piece of paper for the patient to take away.

The Health Education Authority have produced a valuable resource book of educational material designed for ethnic minority groups (see Further reading).

TEAM WORK

The essence of rehabilitation of older people requires team work and plenty of time. Valued additional members of the team may be a social worker or health visitor with specific expertise in caring for ethnic minority patients, and also an interpreter. All members of the team may need to spend more time explaining the aims of therapy and the likely outcome to both the individual and their family. A home visit may be invaluable to set aims and objectives and to ensure that improvement is maintained after discharge. This involves staff stepping into, accepting and adapting their advice to the culture of the individual. A checklist of points for all members of the rehabilitation team to consider is given in Table 3.3.

Table 3.3 Checklist for rehabilitation staff

Communication

Have the following been explained? (Use an interpreter if necessary.)
- instructions about medication
- implications of illness and likely recovery
- need for further tests
- roles of various therapists
- aims of rehabilitation therapy
- follow-up arrangements

Religion

Are there particular religious requirements?
- formal prayer
- fasting

Diet

Are there particular dietary requirements?
- vegetarian
- halal meat

Hygiene

Are there particular hygiene requirements?
- running water for washing
- ritual washing
- use of left hand for toilet and right for eating

Social

Is the patient receiving the appropriate social benefits?
- state or private pension
- attendance allowance
- mobility allowance

COMMON HEALTH AND SOCIAL PROBLEMS

STROKE

Stroke illness makes demands at all levels of health and social service and also tests family relationships, whatever the culture. There are many common misapprehensions about stroke (Table 3.4) which may hamper recovery and need to be tackled. More leaflets and videos about stroke illness in different languages are required. The setting up of more stroke clubs to cater for ethnic minorities may also help. Segregation here may be beneficial due to the language and perceptual difficulties often encountered after a stroke.

Table 3.4 False beliefs about stroke

Strokes are the same as heart attacks.

Strokes are a punishment.

Patients can get better just as quickly as they became ill.

Exercise is bad for the hemiplegic side.

Patients need plenty of rest until complete recovery occurs.

Physiotherapists, occupational therapists and speech therapists are types of nurse.

Treatment of strokes is mainly tablets from the doctor.

Relatives and friends can't help with treatment.

DEPRESSION AND DEMENTIA

Depression may be undertreated in ethnic minority patients, as it is often difficult to diagnose and may present with more physical symptoms. Depression may prevent a patient reaching his or her full potential and may be more readily detected by nurses and therapists who spend longer periods in close contact with the individual patient, than do doctors. Likewise, dementia is less easily diagnosed, as the family may be less forthcoming with the symptoms of personality change and memory impairment. Psychological tests can be misleading, as they are dependent on language ability and educational background. Transcultural psychiatry is becoming an accepted specialist branch of practice (Burke, 1989).

AMPUTATIONS

Leg amputations may be very much less easy to accept in some ethnic minority groups. This is because it implies disfigurement and potential loss of income. Patients may not be aware of the possibilities of achieving independence and a good quality of life following the operation – with appropriate help. Effective counselling and a positive approach may help to overcome these problems.

SKIN AND HAIR CARE

People of Afro-Caribbean origin often use moisturizing cream on their skin and this will need to be continued. Hair care is also a specialized task and should be appropriately undertaken.

RECOMMENDATIONS TO IMPROVE CARE OF ELDERLY ETHNIC MINORITY PATIENTS

The many ethnic minority groups have widely differing needs and it is, therefore, difficult to make general recommendations. However, the following five points should be considered.

1. Teaching about the special needs of ethnic minority elderly patients should be included in the training of all health professionals.
2. More health education leaflets, books and videos should be available in different languages to help explain the facilities already available and their accessibility and purpose.
3. More specialist workers, e.g. health visitors, social workers, speech therapists, community physiotherapists and occupational therapists, should be trained to work with ethnic minority patients.
4. More stroke clubs and day centres, where specific health and social needs can be met, should be for ethnic minority groups.
5. More research, at both local and national level, should be funded and undertaken into the needs of ethnic minority elderly patients and into methods to facilitate take up.

ETHNIC MINORITIES AND THE HEALTH REFORMS

The reforms in the National Health Service following the NHS and Community Care Act, 1990 present opportunities for purchasers to improve healthcare provision.

Historically the NHS was not organized to cater for a multi-ethnic population, which barely existed in 1948. The low uptake of health and social services by members of minority cultures is well documented (Karseras, 1991). The Department of Health has responded to this by emphasizing six key themes that should be incorporated in the development of health policies (Bahl, 1993):

1. elimination of racial discrimination;
2. availability of data on black and ethnic minority groups;
3. delivery of appropriate quality services;
4. training of health professionals;
5. information for black and ethnic minority groups on health and health services;
6. recognition of differing patterns of health and disease.

These six themes should be incorporated in the needs assessment and purchasing plan of local purchasers. However, it is believed by many that the needs of ethnic minorities are far too complex to leave safely to market forces and that there needs to be direct intervention from the centre (Karmi, 1993). The challenge for the future is to ensure that the six themes are acted upon, rather than just incorporated into strategic plans, by all purchasers and providers, including GP fund holders and providers.

SUMMARY

Elderly ethnic minority patients come from widely diverse backgrounds and have a wide variety of different needs. Each should be treated as an individual, but understanding of the various backgrounds, religions and cultures will help to improve medical management and rehabilitation.

Fundamentally the same empathic concern, attention to detail, perseverance and patience are needed as are required to care for other older people. Further research is required into the needs of this important and increasing group of elderly people.

REFERENCES

Age Concern/Help the Aged Housing Trust (1984) *Housing for Ethnic Elders*, Age Concern, London.

Barker, J. (1984) *Black and Asian Old People in Britain*, Age Concern, London.

Bahl, V. (1993) Development of a black and ethnic minority health policy at the Department of Health, in *Access to Health Care for People from Black and Ethnic Minorities* (eds A. Hopkins and V. Bahl), Royal College of Physicians, London, pp. 1–9.

Beevers, D.G. and Beevers, M. (1993) Hypertension: impact upon black and ethnic minority people, in *Access to Health Care for People From Black and Ethnic Minorities* (eds A. Hopkins and V. Bahl), Royal College of Physicians, London, pp. 123–31.

Benefit Agency (1995) *Which Benefit?* Leaflet number FB2, Benefit Agency, Oldham.

Blakemore, K. (1983) Ethnicity, self-reported illness and use of medical services by the elderly. *Postgraduate Medical Journal*, **59**, 668–70.

British Red Cross (1988) *Red Cross Multilingual Phrase Book*, British Red Cross, National Headquarters, 9 Grosvenor Crescent, London SW1X 7EJ.

Burden, A. (1993) Diabetes: impact upon black and ethnic minority people, in *Access to Health Care for People from Black and Ethnic Minorities* (eds A. Hopkins and V. Bahl), Royal College of Physicians, London, pp. 107–22.

Burke, A.W. (1989) Psychiatric practice and ethnic minorities, in *Ethnic Factors in Health and Disease* (eds J.K. Cruickshank and D.G. Beevers) Wright, London, pp. 178–9.

Dawson, A.G., Hildrey, A.C.C. and Floyer, M.A. (1983) Health problems of ethnic minorities. *British Medical Journal*, **286**, 1575–6.

Donaldson, L.J. (1986) Health and social status of elderly Asians: a community survey. *British Medical Journal*, **293**, 1079–82.

Karmi, G. (1993) Management structures for recognising and meeting the health needs of black and ethnic minority patients, in *Access to Health Care for People from Black and Ethnic Minorities* (eds A. Hopkins and V. Bahl), Royal College of Physicians, London, pp. 47–55.

Karseras, P. (1991) Minorities and access to health care. Part 1: confronting myths. *Care of the Elderly*, 3(9), 429–31.

Lawrence, R.E. and Littler, W.A. (1985) Acute myocardial infarction in Asians and Whites in Birmingham. *British Medical Journal*, **290**, 1472.

Norman, A. (1985) *Triple Jeopardy: Growing Old in a Second Homeland*, Centre for Policy on Ageing, London.

RESOURCES AND FURTHER READING

Health Education Authority (1994) *Health Related Resources for Black and Minority Groups*, H.E.A., London.

Hopkins, A. and Bahl, V. (1993) *Access to Health Care for People from Black and Ethnic Minorities*, Royal College of Physicians, London.

Qureshi, B. (1989) *Transcultural Medicine: Dealing with Patients from Different Cultures*, Kluwer Academic Press, London.

Squires, A. (ed) (1991) *Multi-cultural Health Care and Rehabilitation of Older People*, Age Concern, England, and Edward Arnold, London.

...habilitation – ...omplex values of a limitless team

4

Denise Keir

INTRODUCTION

Rehabilitation is too complex a subject to define to the satisfaction of all parties. Descriptions include achievement of, or restoration to, optimum level of ability, taking into account the needs or wishes of individuals and the people nearest to them, whether friends, family or employees of a care service. As rehabilitation becomes a community-based rather than hospital-based activity, power levels change from the domain of the professional to that of the patient. The individual and his/her family carers will be relied upon to participate in the rehabilitation programme and will in return expect to be heard. Such changes will influence the decisions that are being made about rehabilitation plans. David Seedhouse (1988) states, 'work for health is a moral endeavour'. Rehabilitation as part of healthcare then, has a moral aspect.

Consideration of the ethical or moral perspective of rehabilitation requires an emphasis on holistic, person-centred care and the four guiding principles of healthcare ethics (Gillon, 1985):

- respect for persons and autonomy
- beneficence (doing good)
- non-maleficence (avoidance of harm)
- justice.

These are used here to link this concept to professional practice within a coherent moral framework. Inevitably, moral issues arise at personal, team and institutional levels. Rehabilitation takes place in the real world and consideration must be given to the social/cultural/religious practices and conventions of society, rules and professional codes of practice and the law. Britain today is a multicultural, multifaith society and so it is important to consider how the concept of rehabilitation might be viewed from these different perspectives. A problem is likely to occur when the dominant culture controls the legislation and thus the purse strings, influencing how care is provided. Increasingly, too, practitioners are considering how the major ethical theories can help to illuminate ethical dilemmas in this field.

THE PRODUCT AND THE PROCESS OF REHABILITATION

Both the product and process of rehabilitation must benefit the older person. The product is a state of affairs where that person enjoys an optimal degree of well being, viewed from their own perspective. But how are 'well being' and 'optimal' defined, and if communication with the older person is difficult, how can the extent of their goals and those of their carers be evaluated?

The process takes place within a context, and there are a number of actors on the stage. All these stakeholders should be involved to some degree in this process. These include firstly, of course, the older person and his/her carer; secondly, all those professionals and lay people who will be subsequently contributing to the well being and quality of life of the client; and thirdly the funding body. Rehabilitation entails a team of people working together towards a common goal, but both the process and the goal itself are value laden. It is this that causes many of the problems that can arise.

RESPECT FOR PERSONS AND AUTONOMY

The first of the four principles is concerned with being respected and valued as a person; this is essential to human well being. It is necessary to define what is meant by 'a person' for a holistic view of caring demands that a person is viewed holistically. A cluster of features define what we mean by a 'person', but does lack of any of these features fail to qualify an individual as a person and, more importantly, to be treated as one? Do older people seem to lose their personhood in certain situations or in certain people's views? Ultimately an individual's view of a 'person' depends on the values he or she holds. Might this explain why some individuals, especially older people, often get treated as 'non-persons'?

Suppose we 'persons' are defined as 'rational beings with active minds who can make conscious, free choices', and agree that the rational will is a person's most precious possession. In that case elder abuse rightly ranks as a criminal act far worse than burglary. Could the by-passing of informed consent regarding rehabilitation decisions count as a form of elder abuse? Also, when is anyone incapable of making such decisions? It is very much a question of intention and the key point here is 'to what extent is the well being of the older person driving the decision-making process?'

The next major question is: who decides on what counts as contributing to someone's well being? Since the prime aim of rehabilitation is personal well being, it is necessary to examine what is meant by this. If rehabilitation is to involve more than a mere geographical change then the quality of life to be enjoyed by the person becomes a crucial factor. One way of defining well being is to see it as 'the having of achievable personal goals'. Without these, 'persons' are mere puppets. So, rehabilitation can only be linked to well being if it is also a goal for the person concerned.

Abraham Maslow's (1943) hierarchy of needs implies that 'all else being equal, a person is better off and more able to pursue higher goals if basic needs are satisfied first'. These might vary considerably from person to person according to many factors such as lifestyle, physique and culture. Do we often rule out the self-actualizing or higher needs of the older person, such as to be seen as still living an independent life, to be responsible for another, even if the 'other' is a cat or canary, or to leave hard-earned property to their family? An older person's basic needs might include tobacco, alcohol, or the company of pets – things some of us would not rank as a 'need' at all. Equally, an older person may not value a tidy, hygienic home, or even the company of others. We would argue that being able to have a degree of choice is also a basic psychological need. The more self-directed or autonomous persons are, the more they will want to determine their own priorities. Respect for persons is founded on valuing all equally and acknowledging that one person's values are not necessarily those of another.

All of us form our values through social contacts, initially within a family and subsequently through education, social and working life. No two individuals can have identical life experiences, but within a given society values are shared. Within a caring profession there is an assumed set of professional values, for instance to see relief of pain as important. Even then, the carer's values can be at odds with those of the client. A well known story is told about Sigmund Freud, who as an old man refused all medication except aspirin, because he said 'I prefer to think in torment rather than not to be able to think clearly'. Freud was stressing the need for someone in his position to be able to make their own choices, being 'autonomous'.

The extent to which the individual can play a real part in decision making about proposals for or against rehabilitation will depend on the degree of autonomy he or she can exercise. This means how far a person can be self directed – to what extent a free and informed choice can be made. It also raises a question about the degree to which individuals should be, or can be, accountable for their own actions and decisions.

There are older people who no longer seem to wish to be involved in any decision making; perhaps over time they have become conditioned to have this taken out of their hands, but it is still worth showing them that even in this they are still exercising a choice, being respected and having a degree of autonomy.

Autonomy, like freedom, is a relative concept; no-one can be fully free or fully autonomous. The aim of healthcare professionals should always be to preserve and promote autonomy as much as is possible. The way in which this can be done is by always attempting to provide a 'window of choice'. Even where autonomy is minimal, small choices can still be made. This respects the dignity and integrity of the person. Very ordinary persons can still show by their actions that they shape their own lives to some extent. An older person weighing the pros and cons of rehabilitation can surely be a full participant in this process.

BENEFICENCE

The second of our four principles is about doing good. All stakeholders will wish to be perceived as doing good and acting morally, but 'good' is a relative term. From an ethical point of view rehabilitation should be spelled out in terms of benefit to the older person, not benefit defined entirely by others in a paternalistic way. The distinction between 'needs' and 'wants' should be made. Individuals are all authorities about their own desires, indeed many desires remain entirely unknown to the rest of the world, but an individual's needs are not like this. They can be unknown even to themselves and this is where the professional's knowledge and communication skills are so important. The older person envisaging a return to their previous environment can be quite unaware of the new needs they will have once they leave the comparative safety of the residential or hospital environment. The desire to return to 'normal' sits uneasily with the new needs that person will have. The perception of what provides benefit will vary according to the perceiver. The view of the older person and those of the team working towards rehabilitation as a goal need gradually to converge, to give a truly stereoscopic picture of just how the resources and policies can complement the prognosis, and balance the needs, wants and motivations of the older person. As far as possible the two sets of aims should become more or less congruent. Such congruency will take time and skill to achieve, and there will have to be some room for manoeuvre on both sides.

NON-MALEFICENCE

The third principle concerns the duty of the avoidance of harm and is not a straightforward opposite of doing good. This principle, like beneficence, is dependent on the degree to which the person is valued. Like negative freedoms it is owed to all people to avoid harming them.

Gillon (1985) quotes the American lawyer Charles Fried's 'risk budget, whereby people decide (however simplistically) the sorts of ends they wish to achieve and the sorts of risks – including risks of death – which they are prepared to take in pursuit of those ends'.

Is rehabilitation and return home a largely unchanged risk or a considerably modified one? How much modification is of an essential nature and how much is to conform to norms and standards not owned by the returning older person? Making an environment 'safer' might also make it less familiar. The healthcare professional will not want to take risks, partly because the well being of the patient will be uppermost in mind, but also because there is the problem of possible accusations of negligence which might bring the individual, institution or profession into disrepute. The older person may well be taking a risk in having the goal of returning home to a perhaps more hazardous lifestyle than he or she would have in residential accommodation. If it is a calculated risk and is rationally taken it would be harmful to deny personal autonomy on the grounds of purely personal physical safety. To what extent do professionals have to avoid harm to the patient and others, especially, if in doing this, consent is overridden? Informed consent must involve the agreement, acceptance and assent of the client. In addition, it must be made voluntarily and be quite uncoerced; the individual must be sufficiently competent and sufficiently autonomous. This means that he or she must have adequate information, based on evidence not emotion, covering both short- and long-term consequences and be expressed in accessible language on the basis of which he or she can deliberate, having had adequate time for reflection. There are, of course, problems with words like 'sufficiently' and 'adequate'. How much time or information is sufficient? Also, just how competent or autonomous must such an individual be? However, informed consent can be briefly defined as action by an autonomous person based on adequate information. Interventions, or doing things to other autonomous persons without their consent, withholding relevant information and distorting the truth due to them are all threats to autonomy and respect for the person and cause harm. The fundamental principle underlying consent is the right of self determination. If this is the case, how can disregard of this principle be justified?

Professionals sometimes argue that the information is too complex for the person to understand, but this argument could hardly hold, if indeed it ever could, when the issue is the environment in which that person will live and enjoy an acceptable quality of life. To quote from a wise philosopher, 'it is not putting yourself into another's shoes that is morally relevant, it is understanding what it is like for that other person to be in his/her own shoes that is morally important'.

Deliberate witholding of information relevant to decision making is a form of deceit. There is no doubt now that according to the various charters being published, particularly in the public sector (by the police, NHS and GPs) people are entitled to relevant information, which will enable them to make informed choices. But does silence, refusal to discuss, even an expressed wish not to know, or be involved in the question imply consent? In the past this has often been construed as 'tacit consent', but strictly, this is not consent at all. John Stuart Mill (1843) argued for the following principle: 'the only purpose for which power can rightfully be exercised over any member of a civilised community against his will is to prevent harm to others'. Mill did think a person's own good might be a reason for reasoning with him or attempting to persuade him, and the line between this and 'moral coercion' is rather fine. A person's 'own good' is obviously concerned with his/her welfare and happiness. But we do not really need a self-evident principle of non-interference, rather principles of legitimate intervention, rules that distinguish acceptable from unacceptable ways of affecting other people's freedom. This has obvious relevance to rehabilitation.

JUSTICE

The fourth principle is concerned with the equal rights of persons to enjoy the 'goods' of society and to be protected equally by the law of the land. Forcing an older person to leave his or her home because they cannot demonstrate the ability to function independently is a direct physical interference and justification of this needs to be very soundly based. Any intervention occurring without consent can be construed as an assault upon the person. Older persons can be harmed through a misuse of power. It is not a defence of indoctrination to say that people want their minds to be made up for them. Relatives who are unwilling for older members of their family to be rehabilitated, so incurring extra responsibilities, may well be tempted to indoctrinate the older person with persuasive arguments and carefully selected information. For example, they might make them believe that they are more dependent than they might otherwise be. This is clearly harmful. It can be the business of advocacy to counter this danger and it is the business of government in a good society to ensure that there are checks on how power is exercised.

Coercion and deception both cause a person to become an instrument of someone else's will; this is against natural justice. Of course, a person wishing their liberty to be restricted in certain ways does also exercise their own autonomy, if the reasons for doing this are rationally and freely considered. The dilemma of carers is: what is actually in the individual's 'best interests', and does this in any way conflict with the equity, freedom and safety of others?

If an older person is not able to argue articulately and forcefully for themselves and there is a possibility of injustice, then they need an advocate who ideally has no vested interest in the decision making. Healthcare practitioners, especially nurses, command respect and trust. They also have personal access to patients and the public, who believe that they have the knowledge to recommend courses of action. They are expected to give the best possible information and be unbiased. But what does being unbiased actually mean? It means ensuring that the aim of advocacy is to empower the individual, not to persuade the individual to bend to the will of others. Whether people ought to be persuaded and what counts as a genuine claim to providing true information in the best interests of individuals and society at large is the business of ethics. The fallacy of arguing from authority is common – the truth or falsity of a given statement does not rest solely on the authority of the person who makes it. It is not the prestige of an authority that makes a statement true or false, but rather the citing of evidence either to confirm or to refute the statement. Moral questions cannot be settled by appeals to authority and this is especially relevant in healthcare. This is one of the arguments for having an advocate who is independent of the relevant authority.

The function of the advocate is to transfer at least some power back to the patient and assist in pleading the cause of the person who is not sufficiently autonomous to do this independently. The older person often lacks power for economic reasons. The criteria for an advocate can be remembered as the five Cs: compassion/competence/confidence/conscience/commitment (Roach, 1987). Advocacy is justified when there is reduced autonomy, for those who are confused or feel powerless, in fact anyone who cannot effectively act for themselves.

The fundamental principle underlying consent is the right of self determination. If this is the case, how can disregard of this principle be justified? It will now be apparent that these four principles overlap.

CODES OF ETHICS

These provide guidelines for good practice and do to some extent bind professionals to follow them, unless they can justify a different response. The third edition of the UKCC Code of Professional Conduct (1992) contains sections that are particularly relevant to those who might be advising on rehabilitation. In following this code of practice in respect of decision making about rehabilitation, moral dilemmas will inevitably arise. This problem becomes worse as resources are reduced. It is evident from looking at these sections that there could be conflicts of interests where the needs of a patient could put a carer's well being at risk. Codes of practice are not intended to be used as we might use log tables. Rather, they are intended to 'illuminate practice'.

SUMMARY OF THE TWO GREAT ETHICAL THEORIES

This is a very basic outline and further reading is suggested at the end of this chapter.

CONSEQUENTIALIST THEORIES – THE BEST KNOWN VERSION IS
UTILITARIANISM

Actions are right or wrong, according to the consequences of those proposed actions. The best consequences are those that provide the greatest amount of good. But what counts as 'good', and can happiness (or suffering) be measured? John Stuart Mill (1806–1873) insisted that all should be treated equally and that no one man's pursuit of the 'good' should cause harm to another. This, however, proves to be very difficult in practice.

The utilitarian argument is for maximizing 'pleasure' (the good), while avoiding pain. 'Utility' is the factor that is the measure of satisfaction in life. Quality of life is something we all discuss. Would a life that is made as pleasurable as possible and where pain is eliminated as far as possible be described as having 'quality'? Robert Nozick (1974) described a science fiction scenario which could be adapted to the problem of considering rehabilitation and its alternatives. Imagine an older person accommodated in a science fiction environment where nearly every possible need or desire could be satisfied. All sensory pleasures could be experienced synthetically and safely in this environment, which could be regulated to be as stimulating or as tranquil as one wished and only desired things could possibly happen. It would, to use the new technical language of the 1990s, be a 'virtual' residential home. Would a rational older person choose such a lifestyle packed with such ersatz 'quality'?

Most would, I suspect, choose instead to live a more normal life where immediate desires are not satisfied so automatically through the agency of others but where we would be surer about being valued as a person. One problem is that preferences change; we may plan for a more independent lifestyle but when the move is imminent we may resist such an option, from fear, perhaps. Does 'informed choice' rest inevitably on making decisions about what we already know? Many long for congenial company without having experienced it, but we would not say this was an uninformed choice.

Rehabilitation should be geared to achieving a lifestyle valued by the person who lives it, but could we feel unable to support just any choice? Suppose an older person wanted to live the life of a miser, spending as little as possible on the comforts or even necessities of life in order to leave more money for someone else to inherit? This might provide sufficient motivation for the patient to co-operate fully in rehabilitation – but for different reasons from those envisaged by the professional.

At first sight it might seem enough to separate self-regarding and other-regarding desires but our complex social relationships with others make this very difficult. One individual may be significantly affected by concern about being a burden to others, whereas another individual may feel that another should, even at the risk of unhappiness, shoulder such a burden.

Utilitarianism argues for the greatest good to the greatest number, but that this should avoid significant harm to others. Suppose the older person really does just want to be left alone to die? Can we, and should we, respect this choice if we have no good reason to doubt his or her rationality? It is a question of trade-offs of the 'goods' of life. Griffin (1986) compares the ingredients of a particular quality of life to ingredients in cooking: 'we can measure the quantities of wine, beef and onions separately but we can only measure their value to the dish by considering them in various combinations'.

DEONTOLOGICAL (DUTY-BASED) THEORIES

This approach holds that consequences should not be the prime consideration. Instead, moral reasoning should be governed by duty. The concept of duty and accountability is clearly expressed in the UKCC's (1992) code of ethics, and duty-based ethics is very relevant when interpersonal issues are being considered. Immanuel Kant (1724–1804) believed in the freedom of the will of rational beings who would recognize a self-imposed rational law: 'to treat humanity in every case as an end, never as a means only'. Very broadly speaking, this can be expressed as 'do as you would be done by'. This gives one a moral imperative that could govern all one's actions. It is more easily applied as a theory within the special relationship of carer and patient, whereas utilitarianism is more applicable to public policies. Above all, Kant's thinking recognizes respect for persons as a driving force in ethics. He valued a combination of freedom and responsibility. An autonomous person, in so far as he or she is autonomous, is not subject to the will of another.

We certainly feel that we have a moral duty to keep promises and honour contracts, and this leads us to believe that we have a moral right to expect this from others. Kant would argue that all promises should always be kept – but this can cause problems. Perhaps the answer is that we should never make promises that we cannot individually undertake to keep, such as rashly reassuring an older person that they will be rehabilitated, for it cannot be any single person's duty to carry this out. Since any promise or contract imposing a duty on another cannot be valid unless that other person has been involved, such promises should never be made.

Moral rights arising from special relationships could include the rights older people might think they have to be looked after by their own children. Rights could be said to be a function of social systems and some societies might have conventions that would back up such a claim. However, variables could exist that would make it impossible for an older person to have such a right fulfilled. One person could have several elderly dependants as well as a young family and it could be physically impossible to honour all these 'rights'. These approaches – utilitarianism and deontological ethics – have remained the most influential over time.

THE ETHICAL VIEW

Philosophy asks questions about concepts that most of us take very much for granted and ethics, a branch of philosophy, examines the basis on which moral decisions are made and what counts as 'right' and 'good'. In our case this concerns decisions about whether to rehabilitate or not. It involves justifying actions and decision making and reflecting upon them. But moral decisions, unlike purely practical ones, are made relative to the values people hold, and the fundamental problem that is ever present is: whose values should predominate? At first sight this might seem that what is good, right or just is simply a question of 'what I think is good'. Yet we do have codes of practice, rules and laws based on a consensus which provide a framework that we use to help us in moral decision making. Can religious beliefs be sufficient to guide me?, one might ask. The answer here is not necessarily, for an atheist could be a very moral person. The major religions of the world share many views on morality, but there are some significant differences in values.

Consider an occasion when a professional has had to decide what was the right thing to do to promote the well being of an older person. What guides the final decision – instinct, intuition, personal values, religious beliefs, advice from others, guidelines, rules, codes of practice, laws, principles, even ethical theories? For example: an elderly woman has been diagnosed as unable to continue to live an independent life at home. She has been admitted to a residential home and has been persuaded that she is there on a temporary basis for respite care and will be going home. This is not true, but the justification given to the nursing staff is that she will 'settle down' and 'forget about going home'.

They have been instructed to comply with this white lie. Should they? Such issues can generate immense argument!

There will be no rubric or set of right/wrong answers about when to rehabilitate, when it might be justified, or what rehabilitation itself might actually mean for the person in question. What is needed is a very careful examination of the concepts that are inevitably brought into play, concepts such as personhood, well being, autonomy, rights and freedoms, duty of care and responsibilities, needs and wants, justice and fairness, informed choice and quality of life.

THE PROFESSIONAL TEAM

'Respect for persons' is the lynchpin of effective team co-operation and where strong disagreement among committed and informed professionals is evident then it is likely that a clash of values is the problem. Each believes that they are right and, given sufficient information and time for reflection, can still feel justified in their view. What if these conflicts cannot be resolved? Equally there are certain to be differences as to the best interests of the older person between professionals and his/her relatives, who frequently disagree among themselves and with the staff, who will have to provide subsequent support whatever decision is taken. All of them are 'stakeholders' in the situation, all have their own perceptions of what can be done and what ought to be done. A degree of personal autonomy is important to every individual in the care team. In the more traditional and hierarchical structures in healthcare it was easier to pass the 'moral buck' up to the next level, hoping it would stop somewhere. But within an effective team each individual should value the other persons who are, after all, working towards a common goal. This demands qualities such as loyalty and good listening skills.

There will inevitably be times when there will be conflicts of loyalty between members of the caring team and the loyalty to the client. Equally, there will probably be conflicts between the loyalty of the team to the older person and institutional loyalty, when policies do not seem to be operating in the best interests of the individual. Even if the team members are all competent, highly motivated and apparently objective, they will experience tensions caused by these different perceptions. Perceptions of a particular situation can vary considerably; our values and prior experiences affect the way we attend to features of a situation and our expectations about them; this leads to individuals prioritizing things differently. Each one's contribution to the well being of the older person is potentially valuable and a successful resolution of such problems will depend on harmonizing all these efforts.

The very first step on the road to dealing with what is a very complex human problem is to recognize that it is difficult. There are no databases of right answers to consult, as each situation has its own ingredients and emphases. Our education system in Britain tends to prepare us for dealing with fact finding, but ethics is not like that. Beware of the person who never has any shadow of doubt as to what should be done.

As the internal market in health and social care grows, how will it influence values in the future? These are factors that we will have to consider in the next decade, as we ourselves become part of the ageing population.

REFERENCES

Gillon, R. (1985) *Philosophical and Medical Ethics*, Wiley, Chichester.
Griffin, J. (1986) *Well-being*, Clarendon Press, Oxford.
Maslow, A.H. (1943) A theory of human motivation. *Psychological Review*, **50**, 370–89.
Mill, J.S. (1843) See (1987) John Stuart Mill 1806–1873, Utilitarianism, in *Utilitarianism and Other Essays*, Penguin Classics, London.
Nozick, R. (1974) *Anarchy, State and Utopia*, Blackwell, Oxford.
Roach, S. (1987) Caring as responsibility: a response to value as the important-in-itself. Paper delivered at *2nd International Congress on Nursing Law and Ethics*, Tel Aviv, June.
Seedhouse, D. (1988) *Ethics: The Heart of Health Care*, Wiley, Chichester.
UKCC (1992) *Code of Professional Conduct*, 3rd edn, United Kingdom Central Council, London.

FURTHER READING

Henry, I.C. and Pashley, G. (1990) *Health Ethics*, Quay Publishing, Lancaster.
Palmer, M. (1991) *Moral Problems*, Lutterworth Press, Cambridge.
Tschudin, V. (1992) *Ethics in Nursing*, 2nd edn, Butterworth-Heinemann, Oxford.

Psychological approaches with older people

5

Charles Twining

INTRODUCTION

Rehabilitation, like most healthcare, has much to do with changing human behaviour; changing the behaviour of the recipient but also changing the behaviour of family and staff. It therefore seems reasonable to expect that the scientific study of behaviour, psychology, should have something relevant to say to those involved in the rehabilitation of older people. There are indeed many areas of both general and clinical psychology that have specific relevance to helping older people. This chapter aims to identify at least the most important and to suggest how they can be put into practice. Problems of patient distress, difficulties of motivation, family conflict and a whole range of psychological problems can make it very difficult to achieve what the team, older person and carer believe is best.

Normal ageing has effects on cognitive, emotional and interpersonal processes. It makes good sense, therefore, to optimize the effects of rehabilitation of older people in the light of these changes. Appropriate adaptation is not ageist – it is age-appropriate. Psychological effects of ageing are both real in terms of everyday experience, and mythical in terms of many people's attitudes and expectation. Getting the right balance is a challenge to both therapists and older people themselves.

It has been suggested that the application of psychology to healthcare can conveniently be divided into three levels.

1. **Universal skills** – markers of good practice in dealing with people, for example good communication skills. These are relevant to anyone dealing directly with patients.
2. **Specific skills** – may be practised by a range of health and social care staff after specific training, and used to help with specific designated problems; many types of counselling would be examples of this. The training required is likely to be specific to that problem area and

supervision would be required from someone highly trained in the relevant psychological skill.
3. **Specialist skills** – for complex or otherwise challenging psychological problems. They require the breadth and depth of skills that come from a detailed knowledge of and training in psychology applied to health-care.

Psychological skills are useful in helping many people, but only a very few problems require the direct input of a clinical psychologist. Indeed, it will be the exception rather than the rule for a rehabilitation team to have ready access to clinical psychologists, and local criteria should ensure appropriate referral. The focus here is therefore on level 1 and level 2 skills, which are relevant to all team members and can facilitate their practice.

THE PSYCHOLOGY OF AGEING

Research papers traditionally conclude by suggesting that 'more research is needed'. Whilst this is certainly true of the psychological aspects of ageing we already know enough to draw useful conclusions that can guide practical aspects of rehabilitation for older people. Two such principles are continuity and variability. Normal ageing is a continuing part of lifespan development (Bromley, 1990). Thresholds, notably the age at which one becomes a pensioner, are administratively useful, but not based on personal reality. Textbooks and other writings on older people usually pay much attention to the changes associated with age: they tend to emphasize the direction of change, typically a decline in function. They can therefore make rather depressing reading. However, the emphasis on direction tends to obscure the actual magnitude of change. For psychological changes, the magnitude tends to be a relatively small proportion of the absolute level of function; the personal experience of normal ageing is therefore one of continuity. For many variables, age differences (what one observes if today's younger are compared with today's older people) are more pronounced than age changes (what changes are observed if the same individuals are followed over their lifespan). Not surprisingly it is much easier to study age differences, using so-called cross-sectional designs, rather than age changes. The latter demand longitudinal study over many years, at least in humans. There are relatively few research projects that have so far been able to yield such data. Age differences are magnified by differences that are common to whole generations, but not the result of primary ageing in upbringing and other experiences. Thus today's 80 year old will, for example, have had a very different education from today's 30 year old. To understand the effects of true ageing, we must make allowance for this.

Conversely, there is much variability about how ageing affects different psychological functions and how it affects different individuals. Some skills are typically relatively unchanged with ageing, others tend to show decline in most if not all people. One widespread finding is for the differences between individuals to increase with age (Fairweather, 1991). Descriptions of such age changes usually refer to the average for a group of people: some will show a lot of change, others much more. It means that predicting someone's ability on the basis of age is much less accurate in later life. Often for a given psychological function the 'best' older people will be doing as well as the average younger person, the 'worst' are, however, doing very much worse (Holland and Rabbitt, 1991).

Generally it seems as though those with the 'best' initial function tend to decline less. This effect even extends to longevity, since there is a positive correlation between IQ and length of lifespan. This selective survival can significantly distort our view of ageing, especially for the very elderly. Thus a group of men in their 90s will tend to be very special: better than the average of their peers when they were younger and showing less than average decline. It means that even longitudinal studies have their limitations.

COGNITION

Memory is often thought of as the mental function most susceptible to ageing. This may be because normal ageing has all too readily been confused with the dementias; memory loss is the hallmark of these diseases. It is true that memory does change with age, but the extent is probably much less than most people imagine. Immediate memory, that which is involved in remembering what has happened in the last few seconds, declines slightly; whereas in young adulthood, we can remember about 7–9 items, we might find this reduced to 6–8 by our late 70s. This itself has little implication for most everyday life. Where such memory is important, for example in using telephone numbers, there are usually ways of presenting the information so that the load is well within this sort of capacity. This is precisely why telephone companies do not present numbers of more than six digits as continuous strings; they break them into chunks so that all will find them easier to use.

Longer-term memory similarly shows a tendency to decline, but the extent of this depends very much on the nature of the task. Our ability to recall, without prompting, stored information shows a clear decline on average, but recognition memory is much less affected. One explanation for this could be that the effect of ageing is to impair the retrieval rather than the storage of information. It suggests that the information has been stored but not in such a way that we can get at it so easily. It is rather as if older librarians were to become rather erratic in choosing on which shelf to replace returned books. A book on the wrong shelf is more difficult to find when you need it. Also, how we ask for and process information seems to make a big difference to the effects of ageing. Older people seem less inclined to use the most effective strategies for processing and storing new information. They also expect to do less well than younger people and this can all too easily be a self-fulfilling prophecy. The good news is that older people benefit greatly from being encouraged to use effective strategies.

The quality of memory also seems to be affected. In an interesting series of experiments (Cohen and Faulkner, 1989) it appears that older people make different kinds of errors when remembering what has happened. The difference between their memories for what they have done and for what they have thought of doing is more marked. They are less likely to be accurate about the latter. They seem to be more likely to make the error of remembering something they thought of doing as being something they actually did. The effects are quite subtle but can have very real practical consequences. One example in rehabilitation is that the patient and the therapist may give significantly different accounts of what happened on a home assessment visit. If the patient recalls that he or she did something which in fact was only discussed, this may be no more than a normal ageing phenomenon, not the sign of dementia. Another example might be the taking of medicines where the consequences of the thought it/did it discrepancy can be profound. It is important to emphasize that these normal age changes in memory will be exaggerated by illness, distress or other difficulties.

Changes are also found in thinking and language. The most pervasive change seems to be the speed of information processing, which consistently shows decline with ageing. Both simple tasks, such as choice reaction time, and more complex ones, such as processing language, show greater age effects when speed and complexity are involved. Put another way, slowing things down a little and making them easier helps everybody, especially older people. Again, this has very practical implications for the way in which we present information, especially in unfamiliar and stressful situations, such as being a patient in hospital.

The changes in information processing, speed and capacity are also seen in a reduction in the ability to divide attention between two tasks; dividing attention leads to more errors and to slower performance. Distractions are therefore especially disruptive. The change in such processing has widespread implications, because so much of what we do carries an element of time. For example, the changes in immediate memory that we noted earlier could just be the slowing down of processing interacting with an unchanged brief memory store. To keep information in this store you need to go back and refresh it every few seconds; just think of how you keep a telephone number in your head while you are dialling; if you cannot keep going round the loop so quickly, the effect is to reduce your memory capacity. No doubt further research based on such memory models will shed light on what exactly is going on.

PERSONALITY AND EMOTIONS

Personality changes with age fit very well with the principles of continuity and variability; ageing has been described as growing more like oneself. There is some evidence of consistent changes in personality, but the overwhelming feature of personality and normal ageing is continuity. This is therefore the experience of normal ageing: you feel you are just the same person you were many years ago, despite obvious physical external changes.

The changes that are found suggest a slight increase in emotional sensitivity and a tendency towards less extroversion. However, actual behaviour will be much more influenced by extraneous variables. Your health and income, for example, will be much more important in determining any changes in how much you mix with other people. What the findings of personality study and ageing tell us is that we may take very careful note of how someone has been during his or her life so far; ageing alone will have made very little change, and marked change could be the sign of illness or distress.

Health and income are, as mentioned, two of the major factors determining how content one is in later life. There have been many studies of such constructs as life satisfaction, morale and happiness in later life. Clearly these are very important as targets for the rehabilitation of older people; quality rather than quantity of life may be the proper aim. The good news is that most older people are actually happy most of the time. Depression and loneliness are uncommon and likely to be related to poor health, poverty and family or other interpersonal difficulties. Indeed, it seems as though only a small amount of the right quality social contact may be needed for psychological health; having just one person in whom you feel you can confide and whom you feel close to can greatly reduce the risk of depression (Murphy, 1982).

There are no 'right' answers to good adjustment in later life. It has variously been suggested that either disengagement or activity is important to being well adjusted in old age. The evidence is that a variety of styles can be associated with psychological health. It means that, whereas some people need to keep as active as possible to be happy, others can take a more passive 'rocking chair' approach. We are back again to variability as a key feature and any stereotype is going to be unrepresentative.

A number of life events challenge adjustment in later life. Generally they are not unique to old age, but they may be more common and such challenges are more likely to coincide. Examples of such challenges are retirement, long-term health problems, loss of those close to one and having to change where one lives. A simple example of a widowed person being forced by poor health to move to a residential or nursing home illustrates how easily several of these factors can coincide. Sadly such change is sometimes compounded by well intentioned family members who encourage a move too quickly following a bereavement. It is usually easier to cope if such life changes are spread out.

Retirement is probably the most obvious social milestone of ageing. Most people adjust well to this transition, which of course increasingly affects women as well as men. It can give great opportunities in terms of leisure time and having an income for which you do not have to work. Again, the more abrupt the change is, the more difficult the adjustment. In addition adjustment also depends on the position that work held in that person's life and on whether the pension is sufficient to meet the demands placed on it.

Unfortunately, a rapid change is exactly what is expected for most pension schemes and certainly is what happens when sudden illness is the determining factor. Again, the good news is that 90% of those who retire do so without problems of adjustment (Braithwaite and Gibson, 1987).

IMPLICATIONS FOR PSYCHOLOGICAL CARE

INTERPERSONAL SKILLS

A knowledge of the psychology of ageing, summarized above, can be translated into practical approaches to enhancing individual care. Effective healthcare requires good interpersonal skills; these are a necessary component, not a desirable addition. They have often been referred to as the 'bedside manner', usually with the implication that they comprise some innate talent which staff, especially doctors, possess to a varying degree. It has not been until fairly recently that this particular set of skills has been subjected to detailed analysis. A skills model has the implication that such behaviour can be taught and improved through practice. This approach has of course been greatly facilitated by the ready availability of technology, especially video.

The most obvious of such skills is the ability to communicate, especially the skill of effective listening. It is, of course, readily acknowledged that one of the effects of ageing is a decrease in sensory acuity, notably in hearing and sight (Chapter 15). Spectacles actually provide quite a useful, and not too negative, logo for ageing. The use of spectacles is very common among older people and they have the advantage of being marketed to all ages in part at least as a fashion accessory. This is in stark contrast to hearing aids. Like spectacles they can be considered as simply a sensory prosthesis, but their image and their marketing is very different. The feature most often marketed is how difficult the hearing aid is to detect, usually how small it is. Words like 'hidden' or 'invisible' are very much to the fore.

Good communication starts by getting these things as good as they can be and this is especially so for older people, because of central as well as peripheral changes. It is a simple fact that as ageing is associated with changes in the speed and capacity of information processing, it is especially important to start with the best possible input. It has been wisely said that we have two ears, two eyes and one mouth and they should be used in that proportion.

We all use the redundancy or duplication in sensory information to help us receive input. Thus, we all use the synchrony between voice and lips to help get the message across. Compare talking with someone face to face in a noisy room with trying to talk to someone on the telephone surrounded by the same noise.

The rate of flow of information is less if we use familiar rather than unfamiliar language and, of course, if we slow down. This does not mean that we must be patronizing and treat all older people as if they are intellectually impaired. In fact, sticking to the familiar is quite a challenge, because it means starting from what is familiar for each individual, and of course the variability is that much greater in later life. What we need to know is how the individual sees things, what he or she already knows and thus how best to communicate.

Listening to older people is probably one of the greatest rewards of helping them. What they have more than anybody else is wisdom and experience. Again, we note that they are also more different one from another. This means that you will hardly ever hear the same story from two different people. You might hear the same story from the same person. The skill is to use such techniques as reflection and by open questioning to draw out different threads.

Good listening is also essential to identifying important expectations and attitudes. Ageism is frequently to be found among older people themselves. It may be reflected in limited expectations of recovery, negative reactions to suggestions of new learning and other challenges to rehabilitation.

Likewise, families and staff all have attitudes to healthcare that may affect the delivery of that care (Biggs, 1989). 'Ageism' implies a negative, even nihilistic, view of the health of older people. It suggests assumptions about not bothering to provide the best available treatments and other inequalities. Interestingly, such attitudes can interact with behaviour in subtle but important ways in the physical presentation of illnesses in later life. Many illnesses, for example myocardial infarction and bowel disease, have been shown to present differently in later life. For example, a heart attack is less likely to give rise to severe chest pain in older rather than in young people. It is more likely to present by some other event such as a collapse. In general the trend is for disease to present more with signs (that is things that others can observe) rather than symptoms (namely what you feel and tell other people about). Pain is a symptom, a fall a sign. If symptoms are less striking, does it influence how older people or their carers seek help? It may then be that the difficulty that this imposes on the disease being detected makes it more difficult to treat the illness. This can very neatly confirm the view that treatment is less effective in older people.

Services for older people are among those that have been described by observers as 'Cinderella' services, having less status and being less attractive to the most able professionals. This has changed, but the reality is still that dealing with a multiplicity of problems is still very hard work.

Our view of ageing is very likely to be the product of what we have seen. Good practice probably does more than anything else to encourage and attract the most able. Likewise, the experiences of older people themselves will have shaped their views of illness and ageing. Some of those experiences may have been a long time ago. A patient being told that he or she has had a 'fit' after a stroke may carry images of what happened to those diagnosed as epileptic 50 or 60 years ago (Chapter 1). Staff need to understand the individual context to make sense of individual reality.

SPECIFIC SKILLS

There are a number of areas of psychological care in the rehabilitation of older people where any appropriately trained member of the team can provide effective help. I shall consider four examples here, but no doubt others will be familiar.

Grief and loss

Like many other psychological problems in rehabilitation, there is no unique link between grief and loss, and older people. Experiencing the death of someone close to one can happen at any age. What is more likely to be the experience of older people is the cumulative effect of several bereavements, the chance that the lost loved one may have been close to them for a very long time, and people's expectations. There is good evidence that the risk of depression in older people increases with the multiplicity of problems. One of the most important of these is the loss of someone close to them. The relationship may be one that has lasted for many decades. One is likely to be in at least one's 70s before one celebrates 50 years of marriage. That duration may make it very difficult to adjust to the loss, but may also indicate a good relationship. How one adapts is also influenced by the quality of the relationship.

Typical grief has been well described and includes phases of numbness or shock (characterized by absence of feeling or disbelief that the loss has occurred), acute grief (characterized by crying, pining and pangs of grief) and assimilation (gradually adapting to life without the loved one). Adjustment can be a lengthy process and does not follow a straightforward progress through clearly defined stages. This is most obviously seen in how anniversaries and other stimuli can evoke acute grief some months or even years after the loss. Most people who suffer a bereavement do not need grief counselling; they will adapt to the loss given time and the support of those around them. However, specific counselling may be helpful for complex grief, where adjustment is impaired. Factors such as the circumstances of the loss, the quality of the relationship and the availability of support all affect the risk of impaired adjustment. Targeting those at higher risk is the best strategy (Parkes, 1992).

One form of bereavement that could be said to be particular to older people is the loss of adult children. Loss of younger children is rightly seen as a major source of distress. Perhaps it is not always appreciated how important is the loss when the son or daughter is 40 or 50 years old. However, such loss is most definitely seen by the parent as untimely and adjustment can be very difficult.

Disability counselling

In many ways the reactions to disability have much in common with those of bereavement and the work to be done in adjustment is similar. This is especially so in the case of sudden loss of function, such as that following a stroke. One important difference is that disability often follows very serious illness, and in the acute phase life itself may be threatened. There is likely to be pain or unconsciousness and obviously at that time counselling is not a top priority. The point at which it becomes appropriate to focus on psychological issues will vary considerably from patient to patient. It is very often helpful to be guided by the patient's reaction to therapy. Difficulties in adjustment are often manifested as 'problems of motivation' or episodes of acute distress.

Psychological problems are often not raised by the patient directly with the doctor; they are in practice more likely to emerge during a therapy session or when the patient is having a bath. There are parallels with other areas where the patient's willingness to disclose problems varies inversely with the perceived status of the staff member; the consultant physician is therefore at the low end of likely confidants. Often the familiar environment of a home assessment visit may be the best place to start addressing important personal issues. This is yet another example of the importance of team work. A good team enables those involved to share the optimum information within limits of confidentiality, and can identify the best person to help with each type of problem.

Other patients, relatives and indeed other patients' relatives are all potential sources of support, although they can also be the source of misleading advice. Comment or advice given with the best of intentions can create problems when it does not fit with that patient's circumstances. This means that it is important always to try to keep in touch with the patient's view of their situation and to understand how they see their progress. After lengthy rehabilitation, even eventual discharge can be quite threatening. The personal implications of disability can vary widely. Where there is sudden enforced role change, for example, there is likely to be more distress over and above the actual level of disability.

Breaking bad news

Both bereavement and disability are situations in which the professional can find themselves being the bearer of bad news or being asked some very searching questions. It is a fact of health and social care that the least experienced spend the most time with service users, and it is to these people that often quite personal concerns will be addressed. They may have been exposed with some difficulty, and only one opportunity for a response may exist. The response must be honest, and consistent with what other team members might offer if asked. Where issues are sensitive, they should have been discussed openly within the team to prepare any member for such an approach.

Usually we think of these challenges as being associated with terminal illness, especially cancer. However, a question such as 'Do you think I will be able to go home?' can be just as challenging. Like communication generally, it is still only recently that it has been recognized that such skills can be taught. There are several examples of applying social skill analysis to such situations, though usually this has been aimed at medical staff.

All professionals need to be able to break bad news, that is tell patients something that alters their expectations for the future. A common example in rehabilitation with older people is a physiotherapist having to tell a stroke victim that his or her hemiplegia is unlikely to recover enough for independent mobility. An example in occupational therapy might be having to say that it will not be possible to adapt someone's home enough for them to go back to living there. This is very 'bad news' from the patient's perspective.

A useful model for approaching these difficulties and at times painful problems is to view the task as an attempt to bridge the gap between what the patient knows or perceives, and reality. This immediately implies that we need to know both about the reality of future choices and what the patient and family expect. The task is to bring these as far as possible into alignment. At most stages of rehabilitation the focus is on changing the patient's ability or their environment to give the maximum amount of independence. We also need to take account of how much the patient wants to know and how best to tell them. This is particularly important, because there can be a gap, which results in unnecessary pessimism. Realignment of a rehabilitation programme is best achieved with what is seen as a positive approach – focusing on skills rather than failures.

Equally important is to be able and willing to recognize when the goals of rehabilitation change. Generally in the early stages the emphasis is on encouraging the patient and enhancing motivation. We need the patient to believe that all the hard work we are going to recommend in rehabilitation will, in the end, be worth it. The message is something like 'work hard and you will improve'. Often at a later stage we have to change the goals to working to maximize independence within what may be very serious limitations. The message here is 'let's see how we can help you live with your disability'. This change is very often not explicit and certainly the patient may not agree to these different goals. There is, therefore, a dilemma in that at one stage we are asking the patient to put in much effort when in reality it may be very hard to predict how independent he or she will eventually become. Sometimes this is inherent in the nature of the illness (stroke outcome is known to be hard to predict) or it may be because there are subsequent additional health problems (for example problems with a hip prosthesis). Where there is only a rough idea of the likely outcome the tendency is to err on the side of optimism when predicting for the individual – also responding to the need of professionals to feel of value, whatever the hopelessness of the situation.

Inevitably in so doing we may create a bad news gap later on when the individual outcome is not as good as we might have hoped. When patients are discharged from therapy they and their families can express feelings of being abandoned. Sometimes they are sure that if only they could continue having more therapy they would eventually make a much better recovery. Of course, sometimes they could be right, but resources will direct activity to where it can be of most value overall. However, there are also cases where the patient really has reached their maximum recovery and no amount of extra input is going to regain full function. Skill in breaking bad news is very relevant to preparing patients for life after rehabilitation.

Life stories and reminiscence

Thinking about one's past life and telling others about it has been one of the traditional stereotypes of later life. It has been suggested that some form of life review may be a necessary precondition for a happy old age and an important part of accepting one's own mortality. Reminiscence and life review have thus also been suggested as forms of psychological therapy appropriate to older people (Coleman, 1986; Gibson, 1994).

In fact the evidence is rather more complex. Reminiscence is by no means confined to older people. It is something that people do at all ages. It is not a necessary condition for good adjustment in later life, but patterns of reminiscence do relate to well being. There are happy and unhappy people among both those who reminisce and those who do not. It does seem that there is maladaptive reminiscence. Being pre-occupied with distressing memories or avoiding all thought of the past are both associated with continuing psychological distress. This complexity means that reminiscence cannot be seen simply as a good or a bad thing. It is not a 'good thing' which all older people ought to be encouraged to do; there are some people who will be distressed by being prompted to reminisce to no good effect. It is helpful to some, interest-ing for many and harmful for a few. Careful selection and facilitating the exercise of choice by the older person are very important.

The range of experience of older people is a source of considerable intrinsic reward for helping older people. In terms of psychological therapy the richness of older people's life stories offers particular scope for the use of person-centred approaches (Viney, 1993). Such approaches appear to offer useful ways of addressing some of the psychological problems that can arise in rehabilitation. However, as yet we have little in the way of outcome research to guide us.

ANXIETY MANAGEMENT

Old age is not a protector against anxiety, although it is usually the major disorders of depression and dementia that are the targets for psychological therapies. Problems of anxiety sufficiently serious to justify a psychiatric diagnosis have been found in 5–10% of a sample of older people living in the community. Of particular interest to those working in rehabilitation was the finding that the most common cause of agoraphobia in older people was anxiety consequent upon a recent trauma. Thus a significant proportion of the 'housebound' elderly are not limited by physical but by psychological problems. Certainly the phenomenon of anxiety or loss of confidence following the trauma of a fall or fracture or – regrettably in modern society – mugging, will be all too familiar to those working with older people.

Such anxiety may respond to the same kinds of anxiety management as would be appropriate in younger adults. Obviously there is the need to adapt strategies to suit the physical capabilities of the patient. The invention of the personal stereo has been a great help in this regard. It is possible to provide taped instructions as part of a management package at a suitable 'in the ear' decibel level for all but the most hearing impaired. It certainly seems a lot better than having to try and shout relaxation instructions in a calm and soothing voice!

MORTALITY, DEPRESSION AND SUICIDAL INTENT

Coming to terms with the inevitability of one's own death is quite properly seen as a common psychological task for older people and especially for those whose health has been impaired. We know that older people, especially those with chronic health problems, suffer from depression (Evans, Copeland and Dewey, 1991), and we know that this is a treatable distress. There are also data to suggest that the suicide rate among older people is at least as high and possibly higher than that for those in the middle years of life. The rates for attempted suicide are, however, much lower; parasuicide is not a typical phenomenon of later life. Taken together these suggest that we should take very seriously expressions of suicide intention in older people, since any actual attempt is likely to be serious.

Conversely, just to complicate matters, many older people express the wish to die without suicidal intent. Typically they may say something to the effect that they are fed up with living and they will be glad when their time has come. This is particularly so in those whose health is failing, including some who are receiving rehabilitation. Such patients may have a very clear idea of having had a full and interesting life and have come to terms with the fact of their mortality.

Distinguishing between these is clearly important and certainly one of the ways of using specialist psychological skills. One of the important differences is that those who are feeling 'enough is enough' but who are not depressed still find much in the present and in the immediate future to look forward to. They have undiminished interests particularly in such common priorities as family and friends.

There have been a number of attempts to devise simple screening tests for depression in older people and these should be readily available in all rehabilitation settings. They can take no more than a few minutes to complete and provide a rational basis for deciding who would benefit from further investigation.

COMMON CHALLENGES IN REHABILITATION

There are a number of clinical conditions that commonly present with psychological problems as a significant aspect of the challenge of rehabilitation. They can serve to illustrate how principles can be put into practice and how to blend psychological approaches with the others in this book.

Stroke

Any service meeting the needs of older people will inevitably find that it has to help many people who have suffered a stroke. Like so many other conditions, stroke is not confined to old age, but the incidence and prevalence rise steeply with age. Although the age-specific incidence may be falling (the population is getting healthier) the absolute number of people having strokes will continue to increase.

Stroke is a fine example of the factors that can cause psychological distress. It happens suddenly, is not prepared for, can lead to serious disability, has an uncertain prognosis, especially in the early stages, and can affect mood, behaviour and appearance as well as physical function. Little wonder that stroke patients have been found to be at high risk for depression and that psychological variables can play a significant role in how well people adjust following physical rehabilitation. Some of the skills relevant to the psychological aspects of stroke have already been mentioned; the sudden onset of disability can provoke grief reactions, uncertainty of outcome can lead to problems of motivation and coming to terms with significant residual disability can be a major challenge. All of this is compounded by the primary neurological effects of stroke which can include varying degrees of memory and other cognitive impairment. Stroke rehabilitation is an obvious area for deploying psychological resources to the rehabilitation team.

Trauma and orthopaedics

The simple picture of fracture–rehabilitation–independence does not always capture the course for each individual patient, especially in orthogeriatric rehabilitation. The trauma may be the event that tips a person, who was just coping independently with some chronic illness, over the threshold into dependency. The effects of a hospital stay, pain and sometimes isolation due to infection can all take their toll. Maintaining motivation for rehabilitation can be especially difficult when progress is slow and painful. Setbacks in the clinical condition add to the problems. Certainly depression is a serious risk, as is anxiety, and both justify appropriate intervention.

Parkinson's disease

Parkinson's disease has its own very special sort of uncertainty. Despite the initial success of dopamine replacement therapy, we now know that some patients will eventually progress to seriously disabling symptoms, which medication cannot adequately control. In particular this can include physical 'on/off' phenomena and 'freezing'. These problems for each patient can vary not just from day to day but from hour to hour. The effect in terms of disruption of the patient's control over their life is very considerable. Some patients cope remarkably well, but others find the experience leads to a 'learned helplessness' depression. Like stroke, the origin of the disease in the brain makes it difficult for some sufferers to come to terms with the illness. The fluctuations in function can even leave some patients, certainly some relatives and even some staff, thinking that the real problem is simply that they are not trying hard enough. Such thinking can be very unhelpful to rehabilitation.

Memory impairment and dementia

Helping those with memory problems and dementia is quite enough to justify a book just on that topic (Twining, 1991). It is, however, sufficient here to emphasize the importance of mental function in determining outcome in physical rehabilitation. Just as with mood and depression, brief screening for cognitive function should be routine clinical practice in any service for older people. It is important both to identify those who have difficulties, especially those who appear superficially unimpaired, and to reassure those who may be mistaking normal cognitive changes for abnormal decline. It is very important to consider the extent to which someone has awareness of their cognitive or other problems. Cognitive difficulties can alter radically how well someone can manage independently and safely. The level of insight can be every bit as important as the actual level of cognitive function.

Much has been written about memory rehabilitation and the use of memory prostheses. In general the most sophisticated work has been developed almost exclusively working with people with head injuries or other non-progressive problems. The techniques developed work best when other cognitive skills, besides memory, are relatively intact. Older people are more likely to have several problems and require a more pragmatic approach. Simple cues and advice to carers are likely to be of more use than state-of-the-art technology (Chapter 8).

Carers' needs

One cannot exaggerate the importance of informal carers to the successful rehabilitation of older people. There may be many situations where the availability of an able and willing carer is the most important determinant of what happens to the patient.

Thanks to a good deal of recent research we now know a lot more about informal carers and their needs (Jones and Vetter, 1994; Gilleard, 1984). We know that most carers of older people are women; that daughters and sons experience more distress than do wives and husbands; and that many carers experience very significant psychological distress. The causes of this, in addition to sheer physical exhaustion, include grieving for the loss of an equal partner, having to change roles and take on new responsibilities, feeling a loss of control and losing a confidant.

Many carers are themselves older people and the normal effects of ageing apply just as much to them. In practice they are usually a much better example for health professionals of what is meant by normal ageing.

CONCLUSION

The complex interaction between the psychological aspects of normal ageing and disability makes rehabilitation of older people a special challenge. However, the application of psychological knowledge and skills illuminates vital dimensions and enhances the effectiveness of rehabilitation. Much can be provided by members of the team, with appropriate back up from the clinical psychology professional.

REFERENCES

Biggs, S. (1989) *Confronting Ageing*, Central Council for Education and Training in Social Work, London.

Braithwaite, V.A. and Gibson, D.M. (1987) Adjustment to retirement: what we know and what we need to know. *Ageing and Society*, 7, 1–18.

Bromley, D.B. (1990) *Behavioural Gerontology: Central Issues in the Psychology of Ageing*, Wiley, Chichester.

Cohen, G. and Faulkner, D. (1989) The effects of ageing on perceived and generated memories, in *Everyday cognition in Adulthood and Late Life* (eds L.W. Poon, D.C. Rubin and B.A. Wilson), Cambridge University Press, Cambridge.

Coleman, P.G. (1986) *Ageing and Reminiscence Processes: Social and Clinical Implications*, Wiley, Chichester.

Evans, M.E., Copeland, J.R.M. and Dewey, M.E. (1991) Depression in the elderly: effects of physical illness and selected social factors. *International Journal of Geriatric Psychiatry*, **6**, 787–95.

Fairweather, D.S. (1991) Ageing as a biological phenomenon. *Reviews in Clinical Gerontology*, **1**, 3–16.

Gibson, F. (1994) *Reminiscence and Recall: A Guide to Good Practice*, Age Concern, London.

Gilleard, C.J. (1984) *Living with Dementia: Community Care of the Elderly Mentally Infirm*, Croom Helm, London.

Holland, C.A. and Rabbitt, P. (1991) The course and causes of cognitive change with advancing age. *Reviews in Clinical Gerontology*, **1**, 81–96.

Jones, D.A. and Vetter, N.J. (1994) A survey of those who care for the elderly at home: their problems and their needs. *Social Science and Medicine*, **19**, 511–14.

Murphy, E. (1982) The social origins of depression in old age. *British Journal of Psychiatry*, **141**, 135–42.

Parkes, C.M. (1992) Bereavement and mental health in the elderly. *Reviews in Clinical Gerontology*, **2**, 45–51.

Twining, T.C. (1991) *The Memory Handbook*, Winslow Press, Bicester.

Viney, L.L. (1993) *Life Stories: Personal Construct Therapy with the Elderly*, Wiley, Chichester.

Team working in rehabilitation

6

Margaret Hastings

The process of rehabilitation has been described as 'continuous and multifactorial ... dependent on multiple inputs' (Squires, 1993). These inputs are linked through working closely together and sharing knowledge and skills with all those concerned with the patient's management and support. This is essential for rehabilitation to be effective, efficient and acceptable to the patient.

WHAT IS A TEAM?

Concepts of teams and team working vary widely within health and social services and the business sector. Definitions of a team may vary from a group of people working together, to a specific number of people who share their expertise, organizing themselves purposefully to accomplish shared goals. Characteristics of a team are described by Caird *et al.* (1994) as follows.

- The team has two or more members.
- Members contribute their skills within interdependent roles towards shared goals.
- Team identity is distinct from individual members' identities.
- There are established methods of communicating within the group and with other teams.
- The structure is explicit, task and goal orientated, organized and purposeful.
- The effectiveness of the team is reviewed periodically.

Rehabilitation requires a range of competencies and expertise not available from any one individual member of the team. It also requires staff from different agencies, e.g. health service, social service and voluntary agencies, to work together. The tasks and goals set by the team could not be achieved by individuals alone, due to time and resource constraints, and no individual can possess all the relevant competencies and capabilities. Lewis (1992) identified four aspects of a team that indicate the breadth of skills needed.

1. Adapting to the environment and utilizing organizational resources effectively, in order to satisfy the requirements of the team sponsor.
2. Relating effectively with people outside the team, in order to meet the needs of the consumer, whether internal or external to the organization.
3. Using systems and procedures appropriately to carry out goal orientated tasks.
4. Working in a way that makes people feel part of the team.

THE VALUE OF TEAM WORK

The skills required for effective team working can be learned and developed, to ensure that the sum of the parts of the team is greater than the whole. Above all, it involves trust, knowledge and effective communication skills. Team working is most valuable when staff have to work together with a common purpose to achieve a consistent quality of service within the resources available. A well managed team will work effectively and efficiently, ensuring that resources (mainly costly professional time) are used appropriately. There will be transfer and sharing of skills to ensure that patients' needs are met and provider and service user time is not wasted.

In the continually changing health and social care sector, effective and flexible team working will be essential in sharing the workload to meet deadlines and to provide support to team members. Much psychosocial and physical support will be provided within effective team working, for the stresses individuals face when working in vulnerable situations, such as in isolation; with emotive problems, e.g. working with Alzheimer's patients; and in high-risk areas, e.g. community rehabilitation in an area of social deprivation and high addiction rate.

GROUPS OR TEAMS?

The variety of the tasks within rehabilitation will require different problems to be addressed by either groups or teams. Groups will work best for short-term specific tasks. Team work is more appropriate where there is a need for staff to work together towards a common purpose. Team working will be more costly in resource terms, with staff requiring time to meet together to plan, negotiate and share a common purpose. It will take longer to make decisions, with increased discussion and problem analysis from a well structured team. For some tasks within rehabilitation, e.g. the design of a basic referral form, it may be more effective to use a group for decision making rather than the full team. The following chart suggests the factors that affect the choice of working in groups or teams (Henderson *et al.*, 1994).

When to use groups	When to build teams
Simple tasks or 'puzzles'	Highly complex tasks or problems
Co-operation sufficient	Consensus essential
Minimum discretion	High level of choice and uncertainty
Fast decision needed	High commitment needed
Few competencies required	Broad range of competencies required
Members' interests inherently conflicting	Members' individual objectives can motivate
Organization credits individuals for operational outputs	Organization rewards teams for strategy and vision building
Innovative responses sought	Balanced views sought

TEAM FORMATION

There are many instances in health and social services where groups of people have historically arrived together to form a team, without the necessary organizational structure. They have sometimes evolved into chaos, where conflict, differing values and interpersonal difficulties have reflected poorly on the team work philosophy, or, by pure luck, have found common ground and solved the problem.

Health and social care workers are likely to be members of several different teams:

- intra-professional team (own profession with peer support);
- inter-professional team (patient-focused care);
- project team (specific development or management function).

The individual expectations of, and contributions to, each team will vary but all teams will require a variety of tasks to be performed within the team and to develop through the stages of team building. All teams require to have an organizational structure defined which provides an environment that will survive the inevitable changes in membership and demands (Ovretveit, 1994). Within health and social care, team work skills need to be learned, and all new members of a 'team' need development to enable them confidently and effectively to fulfil their team role.

TEAM ROLES

No one team member can possibly be expected to have all the necessary competencies to perform the key skills. Each member must identify their own strengths and weaknesses and know the roles in which they are most competent. Belbin (1993) has identified eight roles for team members. Those required in each team will depend on the task to be performed.

- **The Implementer** Disciplined, reliable, conservative and efficient. Turns ideas into practical actions. *Weaknesses*: somewhat inflexible; slow to respond to new possibilities.
- **The Co-ordinator** Mature, confident, a good chairperson. Clarifies goals, promotes decision making, delegates well. *Weaknesses*: can be seen as manipulative; delegates personal work.
- **The Shaper** Challenging, dynamic, thrives on pressure. Has the drive and courage to overcome obstacles. *Weaknesses*: can provoke others; hurts people's feelings.
- **The Plant** Creative, imaginative, unorthodox. Solves difficult problems. *Weaknesses*: ignores details; too preoccupied to communicate effectively.
- **The Resource Investigator** Extrovert, enthusiastic, communicative. Explores opportunities. Develops contacts. *Weaknesses*: over-optimistic; loses interest once initial enthusiasm has passed.
- **The Monitor–Evaluator** Sober, strategic and discerning. Sees all options. Judges accurately. *Weaknesses*: lacks drive and ability to inspire others; overtly critical.
- **The Team Worker** Co-operative, mild, perceptive and diplomatic. Listens, builds, averts friction, calms the waters. *Weaknesses*: indecisive in crunch situations; can be easily influenced.
- **The Completer–Finisher** Painstaking, conscientious, anxious. Searches out errors and omissions. Delivers on time. *Weaknesses*: inclined to worry unduly; reluctant to delegate; can be a nit-picker.

Everybody will play several roles to a varying degree. Group roles can be learned by observation and practice, and behaviour can be constrained and modified. Belbin's recommendation to individuals is to perfect the team roles already held; work at those that are weaker, to hold in reserve; and forget those that feel unnatural.

All members of a multidisciplinary rehabilitation team will also have a specialist role in their own area of clinical expertise. Within a well developed and balanced team, where trust has evolved, there will be a willingness to share professional skills among team members.

Demarcation disputes over professional boundaries are less likely to arise and there will be more flexibility of roles at times of increased pressure, to enable the task to be performed.

STAGES OF TEAM DEVELOPMENT

Bion (1961) and Tuckman (1965) have modelled four stages of team development, each having four dimensions that need attention: group behaviour, group tasks or issues, interpersonal skills and leadership.

FORMING STAGE

At this stage the team is in its infancy and members need to come together before any output can be achieved.

Group behaviour likely to be superficial, with polite ambiguity and confusion. Compatibility amongst team members and linking of people with similar needs will be evident.

Group tasks or issues establish the basic criteria for membership. Orientation and introductions within the team and the role of the team is defined.

Interpersonal skills Safe patterns of interaction are established and inclusion criteria are evaluated.

Leadership The crucial role at this stage is to focus on team members' needs of getting to know one another and clarifying the goals, roles, responsibilities and procedures that are relevant to the team's role.

STORMING STAGE

This can be likened to adolescence and is a vital stage of development to deal with power and decision making. Unless this stage is recognized and the unpleasantness tolerated, the team will not move on to the productive stages.

Group behaviour Operating rules are established and order is created. There will be attack on the leadership which can be emotionally charged in response to the demands of the task.

Group task issues Power and influence issues need to be identified, together with agreement of the decision-making process within the team.

Interpersonal skills Members work through their own control needs, to regain their individuality, power and influence, and thus achieve a sense of direction and purpose with which they are comfortable.

Leadership issues need to be resolved by listening, providing feedback and encouraging working towards shared goals. Conflict needs to be recognized and managed, to clear the air and help the team to become more cohesive.

NORMING STAGE

The team becomes a cohesive unit and begins to negotiate roles and processes for achieving its task.

Group behaviour There is now cohesion and negotiation.

Group task issues Functional relationships are being built. There is a readiness to tackle tasks.

Interpersonal skills There is affection, sharing of insight and recognition of individual skills.

Leadership This ensures cohesiveness and the interdependence of individual members on the team's purpose and values.

PERFORMING STAGE

This stage sees achievement of tasks within the team in an effective and efficient manner.

Group behaviour Growth and insight lead to meaningful functional relationships and collaboration in performing tasks.

Group task issues There is group identify and a recognition of factors that contribute to or hinder success. This is productive.

Interpersonal skills There is trust and collaborative working.

Leadership There is evaluation of team work and recognition of team effort, rather than individual efforts, to avoid disruption, competitiveness and hostility.

Teams will need to recycle back through various stages as the team changes with new members, new leadership and differing roles. Where problems are developing within the team, it may be that one stage has not been properly addressed and the process needs to be revisited, to allow the performing stage to be reached.

All teams will eventually complete their task and need to be transformed. This may be by redefinition, by establishing a new purpose or structure; or by disengagement or termination. Successful teams will try and stay together to retain the strong bonds within the team, but the team must be allowed to disengage and its members accept the different challenges ahead.

OBJECTIVES AND TEAM GOALS

For effective team building, the role of the team should first be identified together with the competencies required to achieve the goals. This will lead to the production of a team specification, which will identify the team roles needed together with the likely membership size, lifespan, objectives and review plans. Any team should exist for only as long as the need is evident. Staff should be appointed to the team who have the necessary skills or are willing to develop these competencies. When team members change, it is an ideal opportunity to review the objectives and competencies required, before appointing new members. This is the theory, but few job descriptions yet identify team roles and interdisciplinary working as required competencies in the rehabilitation field.

All team members must know what the team goals and objectives are. They should be discussed and formally recorded and review dates set.

It is important to make sure that all new team members have the objectives and goals explained to them from the start to integrate them into the team and ensure their effective working.

PURPOSE

This should be specific with a defined role, e.g. 'To provide a quality rehabilitation service to the patients in the rehabilitation unit'. The defined purpose of the team will allow the necessary processes to achieve this purpose to be agreed. The required process for any service delivery will have inputs and outcomes (Figure 6.1), and the advantages of a team-based approach to defining and reviewing such issues will meet purchasers' interest in contracting for processes or protocols of care.

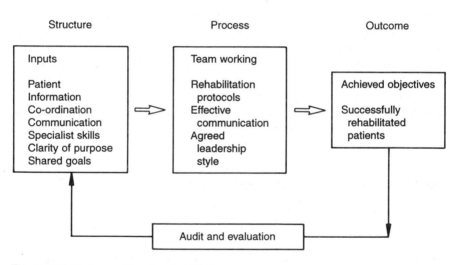

Figure 6.1 Team working in rehabilitation.

PROTOCOLS

Protocols are mechanisms for improving the quality of care. They help staff concentrate on the potential benefits and hazards of an intervention and the evidence on which decisions to use the intervention are based. The Royal College of Nursing (1993) describes protocols as 'an agreement to a particular sequence of activities that assist health care workers to respond consistently in complex areas of clinical practice'.

Dukes and Stewart (1993) suggest that protocols make implicit practice explicit. Protocols are derived from clinical guidelines, which are 'systematically developed statements which assist in decision making about appropriate health care for specific conditions' and are research based. Protocols are an 'adaptation of a clinical guideline to meet local conditions and restraints' (Clinical Resource and Audit Group, 1993). They should be realistic, given local practice and resources, and should reflect national standards of professional practice (Figure 6.2).

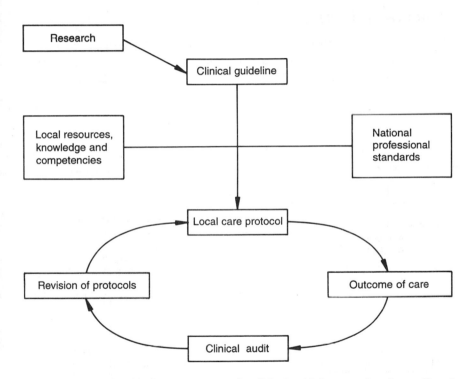

Figure 6.2 Relationship between research, clinical guidelines, protocols, audit and outcomes.

Protocols reflect the process of care within the given local structure. These are essential in specialities such as care of the elderly, where multiprofessional input is paramount in providing care to patients with many problems resulting from multiple pathology. Where multiprofessional protocols are developed, team work and collaboration will be enhanced. Protocols can include:

- referral procedures
- assessment by whom/when/where
- timing of investigations
- treatment plans
- care plans
- drugs
- mobility/functional activity measures
- diet
- discharge planning process
- additional information.

PROTOCOL DEVELOPMENT

Considerable work in this area has been carried out within the UK (at the Central Middlesex Hospital) (Chartered Society of Physiotherapy, 1995). Figure 6.3 suggests the necessary stages over a 6–12 month time scale.

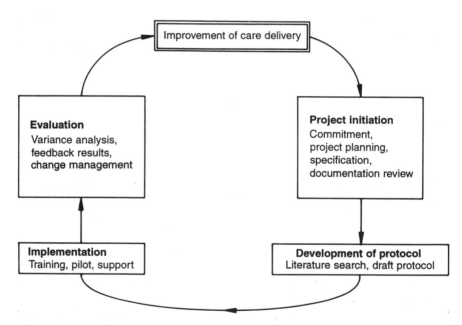

Figure 6.3 Protocol development

OUTCOMES

Figure 6.1 identified the inputs to the rehabilitation team which are part of the structure. Protocols are part of the process, and what results from the intervention is the outcome. In health and social care the outcome is the effect of that care on the user, including the costs of providing that care. 'Outcome is more difficult to define than structure and process standards and is arguably the most important of the three' (Koch, 1991). Increasing emphasis is being placed on outcome measurement and research within the NHS is co-ordinated by the UK Clearing House for the Assessment of Health Outcomes (address given after the references).

Outcomes should be understandable to the patient as the expected result of the care package. If the care package is for rehabilitation of an elderly patient, then the outcome must be achievement of agreed functional goals, to maintain optimal quality of life in the chosen environment. Inexperienced clinicians may fall into the trap of assuming outcomes always to reflect a forward progression in ability, but maintenance of a functional level or adequate pain control in a deteriorating condition are equally acceptable outcomes, and should be recorded as such (see also Chapter 5).

SKILL IDENTIFICATION

In setting up a new multidisciplinary team the objectives and goals of the team will have been considered and the list of skills required in carrying out its function will have been identified. For successful team working the members will have to contribute their skills and expertise to the team's goals. Not all physiotherapists, occupational therapists, nurses, social workers and doctors are natural team members, although they may have the necessary client-based skills. In a career in rehabilitation, especially with older people, these interpersonal skills are essential and can be acquired where there is a genuine desire to learn. All teams will have a mixture of task and people functions which require a variety of skills. Skills found to have a positive effect on team working (Alderson, 1992) are:

- good interpersonal relationships, with understanding of each other's value and management style;
- the ability to discuss issues openly without arousing undue sensitivity or tension;
- a high level of trust in each other;
- being approachable and able to accept objective feedback and criticism;
- sufficient discipline and cohesion to implement agreed decisions;
- the capacity to discuss and understand both long- and short-term issues.

MEETINGS

In rehabilitation of older people, two types of team meetings will be required:

- *Patient-specific meetings* – where all team members contribute to the discussion on the patient's progress, identifying goals and their achievement and planning discharge. The patient's problems will need to be considered from a psychosocial model, not solely a medical model.
- *Team performance meetings* – where the structure, objectives, goals, policies and strategies can be discussed and the team performance evaluated.

For the team meeting to be a valuable use of time, everybody attending should know the purpose of the meeting and what contribution they are expected to make. Standard formats for patient meetings should be followed and an agenda circulated for all other meetings. An agreed method of recording decisions and actions to be taken, by whom and when, must be made and adhered to. This record should be auditable.

CONFLICT

Teams that are in total harmony and avoid conflict will not work effectively, as the team will be working in a closed system and encouraging 'group think' (Ovretveit, 1994). Multidisciplinary teams bring together different perspectives and skills in a co-ordinated manner to provide for the needs of the individual patient. Conflict and differences are to be expected and need to be handled positively for the good of the patient and the creativity of the team. Areas of possible conflict identified within multidisciplinary teams are role ambiguity, role conflict and role overload due to different professional expectations (Embling, 1995). Where role and hierarchy cultures are dominant within an organization, conflict will be prevalent. Supportive and achieving cultures will encourage service user rather than role focus and reward defective teams (Harrison, 1987). Sharing roles and trusting other team members to represent other professions appropriately shows maturity and support within a team. This can be particularly difficult for recently qualified professionals still learning their own role and concerned about who is to carry out different tasks. It will be recognized in mature teams that a representative can only report what they have been briefed on, and will need to recognize their need to seek out further information and report back if the answer to a problem is not known.

Decision-making processes must be identified and agreed within the team. Ovretveit (1994) identifies four types of decision which reflect on the team members and their level of management accountability.

1. profession-specific decisions about patients – confidence needed in professional role;
2. care management decisions about one patient – knowledge and experience of local situation and/or alternative actions;
3. policy and management decisions about how all patients will be served and about how care co-ordination will be achieved – ability to carry out any changes required;
4. planning decisions – what level of authority is required to implement the change process. Do all members of the team have the same level of authority?

The size of teams will also affect the level of conflict. The larger the team the more chances of interpersonal conflict and the less chance of consensus in decision making. Hellriegel, Slowm and Woodman (1989) have identified some possible effects of group size in group processes and suggest that the teams should contain no more than 12 members. Larger teams will perform better by restructuring into smaller groups to achieve the team goals. The ideal team is one that is as small as possible, but that encompasses all the expertise required to meet the team goals.

MANAGEMENT OF THE TEAM

Teams will founder when they lose their sense of purpose and objective. Perhaps the time has come to disengage or realize that objectives have never been clearly set. All teams must take time to explore their vision and sense of purpose and analyse the tasks they have to complete within the timescale. The team leader will have to allow time for this and ensure that all team members feel supported enough to be able to share their views. Within rehabilitation of older people the task may be to enable the patient to reach the optimal functional level to return home. With the decreased length of in-patient stay that objective may change, and the required functional level at discharge may be lower, resulting in increased demands on rehabilitation services in the community, to enable further function to be reached. It is likely that the skill mix of community-based teams will change as more unqualified support workers will help to provide the care. Such workers bring different values (Chapter 4), and different roles will be expected of them as team members. It is unwise to translocate a hospital-based team into the community without providing the opportunity to develop the required competencies in sharing clinical skills with support workers and carers.

The level of staff required to join the team will also vary between agencies and on the issues, e.g. policy making, budget control. This can lead to problems where certain team members are unable to make a decision without referring to a higher authority and can be very frustrating to more autonomous members. There may also be tensions between different organizational cultures, e.g. encouraging total personal choice in social services and providing suggestions of appropriate behaviour in healthcare. Is the patient allowed to stay in bed all day from personal choice or should he/she be encouraged to get up and sit in the chair to prevent pressure sores and flexion contractures, and facilitate mobility? For a quality approach, patient choice is essential, but it must be informed choice based on evidence not emotion (see also Chapter 4).

Increasing competition within health and social care is leading to several providers offering similar services, allowing purchasers to choose the provider of the service, with no guarantee that the contract will go in a traditional direction. Team members should bench mark competing services and note what they can do to ensure that their service best meets the patients needs. When services are appointed, there will exist a need for them to communicate between each other – especially if they are new entrants, or where contract requirements have changed. Details and relationships will need to be shared to ensure that the patient, team and purchaser obtain maximum advantage from the new arrangements.

REVIEW

Membership of multidisciplinary rehabilitation teams is continually changing, due to variations in contracts, personnel, management structures and needs of the care group. Patient demography in rehabilitation wards has changed over the past 10 years with older, frailer patients now being rehabilitated in hospital and fitter patients rehabilitated in the community. The decreased length of stay for acute in-patient care also has great effects on the rehabilitation process and the speed with which intervention is required. Even when there has been little change in the membership of the team, it is necessary to review the team to ensure that it has not become stagnant and closed. For these reasons, regular reviews of the team need to be carried out. Areas to be considered are:

- team objectives
- team goals and time scales
- team values
- skills required to perform the task
- staff development

- leadership role
- team effectiveness.

TEAM WORK IN PRACTICE

Joining an established team can cause anxiety, but consideration and development of appropriate competencies can make the process more effective and enjoyable. An objective analysis of the situation can be enlightening.

PROFESSIONAL COMPETENCIES

Are members sure what their professional role in this area is? Are there specific competencies they need to have, such as assessment skills or neurological rehabilitation skills? Do they know which validated tools to use? What specific skills is each contributing that no other team member can provide? Which skills overlap with those of other team members; which can be shared? Are there tasks which can be delegated? Are there any skills that need to be developed? Are participants aware of the current research in the field? Are individuals able to justify their decisions objectively and assertively, without using aggression?

STRENGTHS

What are individuals' preferred team roles? Which ones need to be cultivated? Which ones will be ignored, and which ones will never be achieved? Do such decisions leave role gaps to be filled? Have participants increased their knowledge about the objectives and goals of the team? Are individuals prepared to share their weaknesses with other team members? Is the culture of the team supportive enough for each to share these weaknesses?

INTERPERSONAL SKILLS

Effective communication among all members of the team is essential for successful team working. Time must be taken to ensure that communication systems are appropriate, utilized and functioning. There will be the written communication of record keeping and the verbal (and non-verbal) communication of personnel interactions.

How is the information contained within the team recorded? Has the team ownership of the multidisciplinary record and access to it when necessary? Does the record meet current professional standards of record keeping or do supplementary records need to be kept? How easy are the records to audit? Can the relevant information be found when it is needed? Many teams have discovered that, following audit, record keeping is highlighted as a major weakness. There should be a record of interdisciplinary problems and goals to be achieved with review dates.

Not all communication is verbal. What about non-verbal communication styles? What happens to the message when someone who normally accompanies their verbal communication with gesture talks on the telephone and the extra information conveyed by the non-verbal communication is lost? What happens when one team member 'talks down' to a new team member? How do team members react to criticism? A knowledge of transactional analysis (Berne, 1966) can be very useful in preventing a breakdown in communication.

The skills of communication that all team members need to have or develop are:

- presenting ideas, information and opinions clearly
- giving feedback
- advising and supporting
- participating in discussion and decision making.

Hidden agendas and conflict are two barriers to communication within the team. Within a trusting and supportive culture, these can be countered. Conflict will always occur within progressive teams and should be utilized to promote a variety of solutions to the complex problems the team has to manage. Members will always bring different skills, experience, knowledge and values to the task. Where this is recognized and understood, respect and trust will develop and the team will develop procedures to face and resolve conflict.

Every team member will have some form of power within the team. Conflict from power struggles may arise and it is important that the leader is aware of any underlying issues. Apart from expert power, dependence power (the power people have by giving or withholding willing co-operation) will be the most important to ensure effective team working (Paton, 1985). Position power of the leader and/or team members will also reflect the complex interpersonal relationships within a team. Power struggles within the team will challenge the leader to facilitate effective and cohesive activity.

LEADERSHIP

The leadership style of the team will have to be on a continuum of behaviour which gets the task done and encourages team building. The power role of the doctor does not necessarily make him/her the best leader of the team. Increasingly key workers need to lead the team, especially in arranging discharge from hospital. The leadership example will depend on the natural style of the potential leaders:

- whether they tend towards an authoritarian or a participative approach;
- the nature of the team – what types of roles the team members tend to adopt;
- power – more responsibility leads to greater authority;
- the structure of the task – the less structured the more participative the leadership style can be;
- continuity of membership.

The leader will need to be aware of the informal communication network, the power strata and the preferred roles and learning styles of the team members. Building a cohesive team has to strike a balance between 'preventing conformity' and 'group thinking'. Ways in which cohesion can be promoted are:

- giving open and supportive feedback, avoiding backbiting and malicious gossip;
- confronting interpersonal problems;
- tolerating differences of opinion and criticism that is constructive;
- allowing disaffected members to withdraw;
- being aware that individual objectives may be distinct from team objectives;
- avoiding blaming particular team members for particular problems.

In summary, good social and interpersonal skills are needed by each member of a multidisciplinary team to ensure effective rehabilitation of the older person. An understanding of the roles, development, purpose and leadership of teams will facilitate success and enjoyment for team members.

REFERENCES

Alderson, S. (1992) *Reframing Management Competence: Shifting the Focus away from the Individual and onto the top Management Team*, paper presented at Reframing Management Competence, November, Bolton.

Belbin, R.M. (1993) *Team Roles at Work*, Butterworth-Heinemann, London.

Berne, E. (1966) *Games People Play: The Psychology of Human Relationships*, Andre Deutsch, London.

Bion, W.R. (1961) *Experience in Groups and Other Papers*, Tavistock Publications, London.

Caird, S., Mabey, C., Adams, R. and O'Sullivan, T. (1994) Working in teams. *Managing Personal and Team Effectiveness*, Open University, Milton Keynes.

Chartered Society of Physiotherapy (1995) Information Pack – Protocols. Professional Affairs Department, Chartered Society of Physiotherapy, London.

Clinical Resource and Audit Group (1993) *Clinical Guidelines*, Scottish Office, Edinburgh.

Dukes, J. and Stewart, R. (1993) Be prepared. *Health Service Journal*, **103**, 24–5.

Embling, S. (1995) Exploring multidisciplinary teamwork. *British Journal of Therapy and Rehabilitation*, **2**(3), 142–5.

Harrison, R. (1987) Organization culture and quality of service: a strategy for releasing love in the workplace, in *What is Making a Difference in Organisations* (ed I. Cunningham) Association for Management Education and Development, Polytechnic of Central London.

Hellriegel, D., Slowm, J. and Woodman, R. (1989) *Organizational Behaviour*, 5th edn, West Publishing Company, distributed by Prentice Hall, Hemel Hempstead.

Henderson, E., Caird, S., Mabey, S. *et al.* (1994) *Working in Teams from Managing Personal and Team Effectiveness*, Management Education Scheme by Open Learning, NHS Training Directorate, Open University, Milton Keynes.

Koch, H. (1991) *Total Quality Management*, Longmans, Harlow.

Lewis, R. (1992) *Team Building Skills*, Kogan Page, London.

Ovretveit, J. (1994) *Co-ordinating Community Care – Multidisciplinary Teams and Care Management*, Open University Press, Buckingham.

Paton, R. (1985) 'Conflict' Units 9–10 of T244, *Managing in Organisations*, Open University Press, Milton Keynes.

Royal College of Nursing (1993) Protocols: guidance for good practice nursing. *Nursing Standard*, **8**(8), 29.

Squires, A.J. (1993) Key issues for purchasers and providers in hospital, day hospital and community rehabilitation services for older people, in *A Unique Window of Change*, NHS Health Advisory Service, Annual Report 1992–93, HMSO, London.

Tuckman, B.W. (1965) Development sequences in small groups. *Psychological Bulletin*, **63**, 384–99.

USEFUL ADDRESS

UK Clearing House for the Assessment of Health Outcomes,
National Health Service Management Executive,
Quarry House,
Leeds.

Assessment, goal setting and outcomes in rehabilitation

7

Anna Smith

ASSESSMENT IN HEALTHCARE

Assessment is defined as 'a continuous process by which the acquisition of relevant, quantified and other data will result in the formulation of treatment plans relating to goals which have been actively set with the patient' (Chartered Society of Physiotherapy, 1990). The British Geriatrics Society (Hodkinson, 1981) describes geriatric medicine as 'the branch of general medicine concerned with the clinical, preventative, remedial and social aspects of illness in the elderly', indicating the comprehensive nature of this field and the consequent need for a collaborative team approach. The team is made up of a number of people (Table 7.1 below) who may be involved to varying degrees in contributing to a comprehensive assessment.

For the doctor, the assessment will, in addition to the comprehensive clinical overview for which he/she is accountable, entail precision in medical diagnosis, specific attention to those clinical domains which influence function (e.g. locomotor system), as accurate an estimate of overall prognosis for recovery as possible and the necessary interaction with the patient and carers to respond to their respective needs for advice and counselling.

For the nurse, the assessment will involve the identification of the immediate nursing problems and the formulation of a care plan.

For the therapist, the key components of the assessment will be the physical, social and emotional functioning of the patient.

For the social worker, the main emphasis will be on the social situation of the patient and significant carers.

For other members of the team, contributions of similar assessments will be made as required.

In the context of this chapter, the example of an older person being admitted to hospital as a result of a medical condition is used. The principles that are described are equally applicable to older people referred to a community-based team, which it is envisaged will become more common with primary led care. For the patient, the team approach may become completely overwhelming, particularly if he/she is assessed by several members, all covering the same areas during the first few days following admission. A possible solution involves the identification of a key worker immediately following medical examination, who performs the most comprehensive assessment. The assignment of a key worker is usually determined by the patient's major problem – e.g. for a patient who has sustained a cerebrovascular accident mainly affecting the speech centre, the key worker would be the speech therapist.

Additionally, or as an alternative to the key worker, combined care records are increasingly being used. These are available for all staff to read and contribute to and are kept on the unit. A more recent development is the use of a clinical protocol to incorporate all staff entries (Chapter 5). Both of these methods should ensure that the patient is not subjected to the same repetitive questions and identifies the individual contribution of each team member.

An additional benefit of the key worker system is that through leadership and focus it can contribute to the successful working of a team, and provide a training ground for future responsibility. Walker (1995) suggests that a clinical professional team should have 'little hierarchy yet leadership and a complementary range of skills'. The key worker system allows different team members to become 'leaders/decision makers' and all must be willing to take on the role as appropriate (Chapter 5).

The result of a successful collaborative team assessment should be the clear identification of goals which are consistent with the patient's expectations. Without such an assessment, problems can be missed, goals will not be specific to the patients' needs and subsequent intervention may well be inappropriate and ineffective.

INFORMATION GATHERING

Prior to the actual assessment, team members can obtain clinical details and diagnoses from the medical notes. It is essential for all members of the team working with older people to understand the implications of disease in older people and their altered response to illness. Patients seldom present with a 'pyrexia', because regulation of body temperature is less responsive. Instead, an infection is often accompanied by an 'acute confusional state'. Dehydration can often occur secondarily to the confusion, with resultant electrolyte imbalance. Pain sensitivity is diminished, often making diagnosis, using sensory testing, more difficult. Older patients are also often admitted with adverse drug reactions, due either to changes in absorption or excretion, or to confusion with the actual dosage.

Patients classically present with multiple pathology; this is due to the accumulation of diseases over a lifetime which are often degenerative, e.g. osteoarthritis, osteoporosis, cataract. Other conditions such as atherosclerosis and emphysema become more common with a rise in age. Diabetes, pernicious anaemia and thyrotoxicosis also occur more frequently and the medical notes will provide essential information on the patient's cardiovascular and respiratory status (Adams, 1981; Hodkinson, 1981).

From this information, each team member can decide on the most appropriate time for the patient to be assessed – too soon may compromise the medical condition, too late and the condition may deteriorate and/or the patient begin to fulfil what they assume is expected – a passive role. Different members of the team will assess the patient at different times; the initial medical assessment is usually followed by the nurse's care plan, which is subsequently followed by the therapist's assessments – the latter may in turn influence both the medical and nursing assessments and plans. It is therefore vital for team members to communicate with each other at the optimum time.

Case study	Assessment
Mr B was admitted with severe confusion. Up to the day prior to admission there had been no previous signs of confusion. He was also found to be dehydrated and diagnosed as having a chest infection with an acute confusional state. Following administration of antibiotics, physiotherapy and fluids, Mr B became much more coherent.	1. Medical diagnosis and treatment 2. Nursing problems→care plan + implementation 3. Physiotherapy→chest assessment and treatment 4. Physiotherapy: further assessment once patient is responding to antibiotic therapy 5. Occupational therapy: assessment→function at home 6. Dietitian→nutritional status 7. Social work→discharge planning

Similarly, in day hospitals and in the community it is necessary to determine the optimum time for assessment from the perspective of the patient and from other staff involved.

THE ASSESSMENT

Having selected the most suitable time for assessment, arrangements can also be made, when possible, for the spouse/carer to be present. The involvement of the carer will be dependent on several factors: an elderly spouse may not be physically able to be present, the patient may not be willing for the carer to be present or the carer may not actually want to be involved. The patient may be anxious about the implications of their illness and their ability to cope at home. The patient may find a full assessment fatiguing, especially if concurrently undergoing diagnostic examinations. In such circumstances the assessment can be completed over the following couple of days, although bed throughput pressure may dictate an early and condensed assessment in order for timely discharge arrangements to be set in motion.

The assessment forms a vital part in the development of the patient–clinician relationship. It is essential for the assessor to be supportive, understanding and sensitive to the patient's needs. At the completion of the assessment it is important for the patient to feel a sense of trust in the staff and have confidence that their findings will be acted on.

Considerable research has been undertaken in the patient–staff relationship. For instance, Hargreaves (1987) felt that greater emphasis should be placed on the ability to communicate during training, without leaving it to instinct. Studies have shown that some staff still have negative feelings towards older patients (Finn, 1986), which may influence their goal-setting process (Nieuwboer, 1992). Patients can easily sense these attitudes. French (1990) suggested that a possible way of counteracting some of these negative stereotypes would be for students to acquire knowledge and experience of elderly people who are well. Squires and Simpson (1987) found some evidence of a relationship between the attitude of clinical staff towards their work and the student's own enthusiasm for work with elderly people. One student commented 'the attitudes and enthusiasm displayed by the staff in each area have affected the way I have felt about it'.

SOCIAL SITUATION

Throughout the assessment it is essential to consider all the social aspects and to gain some insight into the interaction between the patient and their spouse/carer. Admission may not have been entirely due to a deterioration in the patient's condition, but also to change in the carer's ability, availability or willingness to cope. The expectation of the carer about the patient's potential or the outcome of the assessment/ admission may be very different from that of the patient, and these differences have to be resolved. The carer's assumption of his/her own physical and mental ability may also be unrealistic and should be explored.

Team members should begin to establish a clear picture of how the patient was functioning prior to admission/assessment, how much support they were receiving and who provided it (Table 7.1), together with details of the type of accommodation (Table 7.2).

Table 7.1 Sources of support for the patient

Psychologist		Social Worker
Dietitian		Nurse
Physiotherapist		Doctor
Speech therapist	**PATIENT**	Occupational therapist
Pharmacist		Chiropodist
Dentist		Continence adviser

Table 7.2 Example of form to be completed on social details and type of accommodation

Flat/house	....
Stairs	....
Location of bedroom	....
Assistance required with:	....
Personal care (bathing, washing, etc.)	....
Assistance required with:	....
Cooking, provision of meals	....
Additional help (shopping, etc.)	....
Social services support	....
Social activities, interests, hobbies	....

PHYSICAL EXAMINATION

A physical examination can be performed when the patient's tolerance allows. If the presenting condition is a hemiplegia then a normal neurological assessment would be conducted. If the problem involves two or more disciplines, such as with swallowing difficulties, it is often beneficial for the doctor, physiotherapist, speech therapist and dietitian to assess together.

The physical assessment is combined with a functional assessment (Figure 7.1). In some units an early functional assessment is made, and

Information / medical diagnosis
|
Interview / assessment
Presenting condition
Past-medical history: Multiple pathology
Social history
|
Specific assessment, e.g. hemiparesis / hemiplegia
|
Functional assessment
|
Problem identification with patient / carer
Current problems
Pre-existing problems
|
Goal setting with patient / carer
Short and long term
|
Recording

Figure 7.1 Functional assessment of the patient.

is used to formulate the care plan. The physiotherapist, occupational therapist or nurse may perform this initial assessment and it should also provide information on how all members of the team can best physically handle the patient.

There are many functional indices in use; probably the best known is the Barthel index (Mahoney and Barthel, 1965). It was one of the first functional indices whereby a patient is observed performing a functional activity and then scored according to whether or not he or she can perform it independently (Table 7.3). It has been recommended as a standard assessment by the Royal College of Physicians and the British Geriatrics Society (1992) and provides an indicator for care levels. In many units all patients are scored on admission and on discharge.

Problems can arise when such indices are used as outcome measures (Smith, 1993) as intervention may resolve a physical problem without necessarily contributing to an increase in functional ability. Neither can such an index measure improvement in quality of movement. The index is not sensitive to change at either end of the scale (e.g. mobility: if the patient is able to walk 500 yards or more after treatment, he will only score 3).

Several other functional indices are in use and therapists often include additional functional measures if they are more applicable to the patients' problems: e.g. the timed 'get up and go test' (Podsiadlo and Richardson, 1991); the elderly mobility scale (Smith, 1994), which includes a timed walk of 6m; or the instrumental activities of daily living (Wade, Legh-Smith and Hewer, 1985), which includes cooking, cleaning and shopping.

Table 7.3 Barthel Index of the activities of daily living (ADL)

Function	Score	Description
Bowels	0	Incontinent (or needs to be given enema)
	1	Occasional accident (once a week)
	2	Continent
Bladder	0	Incontinent, or catheterized and unable to manage
	1	Occasional accident (maximum once per 24 h)
	2	Continent (for more than 7 days)
Grooming	0	Needs help with personal care: face, hair, teeth, shaving
	1	Independent (implements provided)
Toilet use	0	Dependent
	1	Needs some help, but can do something alone
	2	Independent (on and off, wiping, dressing)
Feeding	0	Unable
	1	Needs help in cutting, spreading butter, etc.
	2	Independent (food provided within reach)
Transfer	0	Unable (no sitting balance)
	1	Major help (physical: one or two people) – can sit
	2	Minor help (verbal or physical)
	3	Independent
Mobile	0	Immobile
	1	Wheelchair dependent, including corners, etc.
	2	Walks with help of one person (verbal or physical)
	3	Independent
Dressing	0	Dependent
	1	Needs help but can do about half unaided
	2	Independent (including buttons, zips, laces, etc.)
Stairs	0	Unable
	1	Needs help (verbal, physical, carrying aid)
	2	Independent up and down
Bathing	0	Dependent
	1	Independent (bath: must get in and out unsupervised and wash self. Shower: unaided/unsupervised)

The Association of Chartered Physiotherapists with a Special Interest in Elderly People (ACPSIEP) developed a visual record (Squires, Rumgay and Perombelon, 1991, Figure 6:1) called the General Mobility Index, which includes six activities of daily living. The index combines assessment of key activities with personalized functional goals. It has also been modified for use as a communication chart to convey to staff and patient/carer the patient's progress (Finlay, 1994).

The British Geriatrics Society Report also recommends standardized assessment scales for cognitive function, depression and quality of life, together with screening for communication and assessment of social status, all of which should be available in the notes. The interrelationship between these tests is an area that requires further research.

IDENTIFICATION OF PROBLEMS

Once the assessment has been completed, the team, together with the patient and carer, can begin to identify the main problems. Owing to the nature of illness and disability in the older person, team members may be overwhelmed by the number of problems. By focusing on functional problems together with the patient's own perception of the problems, the team should be able to prioritize them with the patient/carer. This stage of clinical decision making is, however, often dependent on the 'intuition' of experienced staff. Textbooks and research may indicate the way ahead for individual conditions, but this fails when they present in unique combinations. This skill of setting a functional goal from a mix of problems is the specialist skill of those who work successfully with older people. In particular, decisions are particularly difficult when the appropriate approach is not to intervene (Chapter 4), when rehabilitation is unlikely to be of benefit. Such decisions should be made objectively and overtly and they should be recorded. When problems are documented, they are usually expressed as a functional loss, but in some cases the physical problem will be associated with an environmental or social problem. Such problems will involve the physiotherapist and occupational therapist working in close conjunction with each other, and increasingly with agencies external to both health and social services.

Case study

> Mr F was admitted with an acute on chronic chest infection. On examination, he was found to have pain in both knees from osteoarthritis and lower limb oedema; his chest infection was responding to antibiotics. He described his main problem at home as deterioration in his mobility and he stated that he had been sleeping in a chair, because he was unable to manage the stairs. He lived alone and up until the present admission he had been managing on his own with some support from his daughter. His problems are therefore: decreased mobility/ambulation secondary to chest infection and osteoarthritic knees and swelling due to inability to get to bed. He is unable to manage stairs at home.

Rothstein and Echternach (1986) actually make an argument for drawing up the problem list before examining the patient. They stress that the patient's problems are those identified by the patient and 'problem lists generated after physical examination often have departed from dealing with the patient's problems because they have included clinical impressions, diagnostic information or professional jargon'. Most team members will probably continue to formulate problem lists after assessment, but the paper provides a valuable caution.

GOAL SETTING IN HEALTHCARE

As in problem identification, goal setting can be a complex process. Goals must always relate to the older person's expectations. They must be realistic, meaningful, achievable and measurable. Both short- and long-term goals should be set; the latter should be directly related to the achievements of the former. Different team members may initially have different goals and, even when an agreed direction is reached, each may employ different methods to achieve them. Each team member must be aware of the effect their approach may have on others, and be prepared to compromise for the benefit of (the person who matters) the older person. The attainment of goals may be achieved either by a therapeutic or a prosthetic approach (Grimley Evans, 1989). In the latter the physical disabilities are not treated but appropriate aids are provided and advice given.

Case study

In the case of Mr F, his exercise tolerance is decreased due to chest problems and he does not want to travel to the day hospital to continue a rehabilitation programme, because of the risk of further infection. The immediate goal is to improve mobilization, to enable him to go home, by the provision of suitable walking aids.

He would be given advice on the management of his knees; how to avoid repetitive loading of the knee joints, how to apply a cold compress (e.g. frozen peas). He would be taught quadriceps exercises and correct rising from a chair (Adler, 1985). The best method for climbing stairs would be shown, but if unsuccessful, arrangements could be made to have his own bed downstairs with the possibility of an application for provision of a stair lift.

This would involve close liaison between therapy staff and social worker, and with social services for any additional home care services required. A home visit prior to discharge or a visit on discharge could be arranged. The community physiotherapist could be requested to undertake a follow-up review.

Throughout any treatment programme, goals are continually being re-assessed and changed according to the patient's response, both positive and negative (Figure 7.1).

RECORD KEEPING

Many units employ a problem-orientated record format (POMR), which has previously been well described (e.g. Coates and King, 1982). All POMRs consist of a database, a problem list, an initial plan and progress notes. Information is recorded in the database section; a problem list is drawn up; all problems are numbered – this number remains the same throughout. The goals and plan of treatment are included in the initial plan. The progress notes are written up in the SOAP format:

S = Subjective: all the patient tells the therapist
O = Objective: all measurable data
A = Assessment: updated objectives of treatment
P = Plan: any changes in the initial plan.

The data should be entered in such a way as to facilitate the collection of information for audit purposes: e.g. number of times reviewed by team members; whether goals are achieved. Some staff find the use of SOAP progress notes cumbersome and although adhering to problem orientated records, they have adapted the record sheet to meet their needs, especially where interdisciplinary records are kept.

OUTCOME MEASURES IN HEALTHCARE

Considerable controversy exists around the whole area of suitable outcome measures. As previously stated, staff feel that the effect of their intervention cannot be easily quantified on a standard functional index and have investigated alternatives such as problem resolution. For example (Wagstaff, 1994):

1. problem deteriorated
2. no change in problem
3. maintenance achieved
4. problem resolving
5. problem resolved

It is felt that such a score will have some relevance to those interventions which largely involve advice and/or handling skills for the carer. The General Mobility Index allows for compliance with personalized goals, which take into consideration both anticipated deterioration and increasing assistance. An additional problem in a team setting is the collection of single discipline outcome measures which for purchasers' purposes provides very disjointed information. Wider health status measures such as the Nottingham Health Profile have been used in an attempt to assess the overall impact of intervention. The Nottingham Health Profile measures perceived or subjective health status (Hunt, 1986).

Enderby (1992) has developed a measure that combines any change in the physical condition with the level of distress a patient is experiencing. She has proposed using outcome measures based on those of the World Health Organization (WHO) of impairment, disability and handicap, where:

Impairment   =   loss or abnormality of physiological or anatomical structures;

Disability   =   loss in functional performance;

Handicap   =   disadvantage experienced by the individual as a result of impairments and disability.

The measure was originally developed on speech therapy patients, but has now been adapted for physiotherapy (Enderby and Kew, 1995).

In the case of a patient with a fractured neck of femur, the impairment is the fracture, the disability is the inability to walk and the handicap is the inability to get out and socialize. Each is scored 0–5 for impairment:

0 = Severe level of impairment;
1 = Severe/moderate level of impairment;
2 = Moderate level of impairment;
3 = Moderate/slight level of impairment;
4 = Slight level of impairment;
5 = No impairment.

Similar scores are assigned to disability and handicap and an additional score of distress has been included. The scales provide outcome measures that can accommodate a wider range of therapy interventions.

In most departments outcome measures are recorded on computerized systems to facilitate access and retrieval. One package is the TELER system (Le Roux, 1993), which is concerned with measuring outcomes from a dynamic treatment delivery process. Individualized goals are set and the system can trace changes in the patient's ability in achieving the goals.

Additional outcome measures which may be in use on various units and with which all staff can be involved are those measuring satisfaction with care (Royal College of Physicians, 1994) and the degree of strain on the carer (Robinson, 1983). For the former, a neutral person not involved with the provision of care administers the questionnaire.

CONCLUSION

Multidisciplinary assessment is the key to the formulation of shared goals and consistent treatment plans acceptable to the patient and his/her carer. Evidence of the outcome of the assessment process will be increasingly sought by all stakeholders. Some of the outcome measures introduced in this chapter are being used in various units at the current time; there are, however, many more (Bowling, 1991). Staff are now having to make decisions not only on the appropriateness of the outcome measure as an indicator of their intervention, but also on whether it will meet the requirements of their purchaser. Many of the simple standard measures are inadequate because they are only based on improvement in function. In some instances an elderly person will have a chronic deteriorating condition that is not amenable to any change in their physical ability; in these situations treatment will be based on strategies to assist them to cope with their disability. Staff must therefore ensure that the outcome measures also reflect this type of inter-vention.

REFERENCES

Adams, G.F. (1981) *Essentials of Geriatric Medicine*, 2nd edn, Oxford University Press, Oxford.

Adler, S. (1985) Self care in the management of the degenerative knee joint, *Physiotherapy*, **71**(2), 58–60.

Bowling, A. (1991) *Measuring Health*, Open University Press, Milton Keynes.

Chartered Society of Physiotherapy (1990) *Standards of Good Practice*, Chartered Society of Physiotherapy, London.

Coates, H. and King, A. (1982) *The Patient Assessment – A Handbook for Therapists*, Churchill Livingstone, Edinburgh.

Enderby, P. (1992) Outcome measures in speech therapy: impairment, disability, handicap and distress. *Health Trends*, **24**(2), 61–3.

Enderby, P. and Kew, E. (1995) Outcome measurement in physiotherapy. Using the World Health Organisation's classification of impairment, disability and handicap: a pilot study. *Physiotherapy*, **81**(4), 177–80.

Finlay, O. (1994) Communication chart. *Physiotherapy*, **80**(3), 173.

Finn, A.M. (1986) Attitude of physiotherapists towards geriatric care. *Physiotherapy*, **72**(3), 129–31.

French, S. (1990) Ageism. *Physiotherapy*, **76**, 178–82.

Grimley Evans, J. (1989) Curing is caring. *Age and Ageing*, **18**, 217–18.

Hargreaves, S. (1987) The relevance of non-verbal skills in physiotherapy. *Physiotherapy*, **73**(12), 685–8.

Hodkinson, H.M. (1981) *An Outline of Geriatrics*, 2nd edn, Academic Press, London.

Hunt, S.M. (1986) Measuring health in clinical care and clinical trials, in *Measuring Health: A Practical Approach* (ed G. Teeling Smith), John Wiley, Chichester.

Le Roux, A.A. (1993) TELER, the concept. *Physiotherapy*, **79**(11), 755–8.

Mahoney, F.I. and Barthel, D.W. (1965) Functional evaluation: the Barthel index. *Maryland State Medical Journal*, **14**, 61–5.

Nieuwboer, A.M. (1992) Attitudes towards working with older patients: physiotherapists' responses to video presentation of post-amputation gait training for an older and a younger patient. *Physiotherapy Theory and Practice*, **8**, 27–37.

Podsiadlo, D. and Richardson, S. (1991) The timed 'up and go' – a test of basic functional mobility for frail elderly persons. *Journal of the American Geriatrics Society*, **39**, 142–8.

Robinson, B.C. (1983) Validation of a care-giver strain index. *Journal of Gerontology*, **38**, 344–8.

Rothstein, J.M. and Echternach, J.L. (1986) Hypothesis orientated algorithm for clinicians – a method for evaluation and treatment planning. *Physical Therapy*, **66**(9), 1388–94.

Royal College of Physicians and the British Geriatrics Society (1992) *Standardised Assessment Scales for Elderly People*, Royal College of Physicians and British Geriatrics Society, London.

Royal College of Physicians (1994) *Geriatric Day Hospitals: Their Role and Guidelines for Good Practice*, Royal College of Physicians, London.

Smith, A. (1993) Beware of the Barthel. *Physiotherapy*, **79**(12), 843–4.

Smith, R. (1994) Validation and reliability of the Elderly Mobility Scale. *Physiotherapy*, **80**(11), 744–7.

Squires, A.J. and Simpson, J.M. (1987) The impact of clinical experience in geriatric medicine on physiotherapy students. *Physiotherapy*, **73**(10), 516–20.

Squires, A., Rumgay, B. and Perombelon, M. (1991) Audit of contract goal setting by physiotherapists working with elderly patients. *Physiotherapy*, **77**(12), 790–5.

Wade, D.T., Legh-Smith, J. and Hewer, R.L. (1985) Social activities after stroke: measurement and natural history using the Frenchay Activities Index. *International Rehabilitation Medicine*, **7**, 176–81.

Wagstaff, S. (1994) Outcome models for physiotherapy. *ACPSIEP Newsletter*, **September**, 30.

Walker, A. (1995) Patient compliance and the placebo effect. *Physiotherapy*, **81**(3), 120–6.

Mental state and physical performance

8

Rosemary Oddy

INTRODUCTION

The relationship between mental state and physical performance is apparent in many spheres of life: a child's natural physical reactions are tempered by learned experience over time; the athlete requiring his body to be at peak performance can mentally choose to push himself to the limits. The athlete's training needs to equip him both physically and mentally so that he can combine strength, speed and ease of movement with the vital determination to win. The snooker champion's steady hand can be seen close-up on television screens. His superb demonstration of co-ordination depends a great deal on his ability to maintain a calm and relaxed state of mind. The powerful effect of mentally rehearsing any physical task is well known.

Those who have a mentally demanding job and work under pressure are encouraged to indulge in some physical activity in order to 'wind down' at the end of the day. Any exercise increases general well being, and renews mental energy and drive. The ability to relax mentally and physically can be learned; it can be of great benefit to those who are subjected to worries and anxieties during the course of everyday life. Over a period of time these and other skills can become 'engrained' and as life progresses, much of what is done on a daily basis is carried out 'automatically'.

The link between mental state and physical performance can be seen even more clearly amongst those with mental illness. Elderly patients who develop a major psychiatric condition may well be rendered incapable of carrying out the activities of daily living for a period of time, some becoming permanently dependent on others. All team members, professional and lay, must work together, following agreed aims and procedures, to facilitate an effective result. The development of community mental health teams (CMHT) has provided the mechanism for more effective team working, by enabling comprehensive coverage and a co-ordinated response within the patients' chosen environment.

THE AGEING POPULATION

A proportion of those over 65 years develop a mental disorder severe enough to require admission to hospital for care or treatment. Some come under the care of the elderly team; others with severe problems are more likely to be managed by a specialist team. One detailed study (Kay, Beamish and Roth, 1964) found that 8% of the elderly population in Newcastle upon Tyne were admitted to hospital suffering from a psychiatric disorder. Severe organic syndromes, mainly dementias, accounted for 5% and severe major functional disorders for 3%. Another study (Lindesay, Briggs and Murphy, 1989), looking at prevalence rates in an elderly urban community, found cognitive impairment (dementia) in 4.6% and depression in 13.5%. These statistics related to elderly people living at home; they did not include those in institutional care.

CARE IN THE COMMUNITY

The National Health Service and Community Care Act, 1990 laid out the way care was to be delivered in the community and made the Department of Social Services responsible for providing personal services there. The need for hospital beds for acutely ill patients and for some assessment purposes remains, so the success of care in the community depends a great deal on the balanced and appropriate provision of adequate services. The care programme approach (CPA) was introduced in 1991, and care management (CM) followed in 1993. They are similar in structure and provide a framework for good practice (North, Ritchie and Ward, 1993). The CPA consists of a series of formal stages in care planning and aims at ensuring that those referred to the mental health services receive the health and social care they require. Care management is the responsibility of social services to implement and is principally intended for those who have particularly complex health and social needs.

Decisions regarding patients and their care plans usually involve the whole CMHT, as well as patients/carers, as appropriate. Core membership could include a doctor, nurse, occupational therapist, physiotherapist, clinical psychologist, speech and language therapist, social worker and a representative of the voluntary sector. Following discussion of the initial assessment findings by the team, a key worker is allocated to each patient. This person is likely to be best suited to providing the major part of the care plan and is responsible for co-ordinating and monitoring its effectiveness, identifying unmet needs and ensuring that the case is regularly reviewed.

Before the Community Care Act, the more severe cases of depression and dementia were encountered in hospital and the less severe ones at home. As a result of this Act and the provision of long-stay beds in community settings, many people with chronic mental conditions are now being supported in the community. People with severe dementia are increasingly being cared for in nursing and residential homes, but many are living on their own or with family carers, and require a great deal of support.

ELDER ABUSE

During the course of their work, healthcare and social services staff come into contact with many other paid and unpaid workers involved in caring for mentally ill people. They should be aware that such elderly people are particularly vulnerable to abuse (Age Concern, undated). Elder abuse is defined by Action on Elder Abuse (see Useful addresses after the reference list) as 'a single or repeated act or lack of appropriate action, occurring within any relationship where there is an expectation of trust, which causes harm or distress to an older person'. Abuse can take a variety of forms: physical, psychological, financial and sexual abuse as well as neglect. Staff who suspect that abuse is occurring should follow their service's guidelines, so that appropriate action can be taken (Kingston and Phillipson, 1994).

CARING FOR CARERS

Implementing a national policy of maintaining elderly people in the community, including those with mental illness, increases the need to support and train their carers. Lodge (1981) considered that a whole range of services is required for carers, but as yet they have few automatic rights. Forthcoming legislation may rectify this omission and provide some much-needed relief for the millions of devoted unpaid carers who enable elderly relatives or neighbours to remain in their own homes. The Carers National Association (see Useful addresses) spearheads the campaign for a fairer deal for carers and provides them with information on available services.

MAJOR MENTAL DISORDERS IN ELDERLY PATIENTS

Roth (1955) described the categories and incidence of mental disorders in elderly people. He considered that acute confusional state, depression, paraphrenia and dementia were the four major disorders. Most medical practitioners consider the conditions in this order when making their diagnosis. By so doing, overuse of the unfortunate dementia label is avoided, since consideration is given to the other three disorders first.

As an introduction, a brief outline of these four conditions follows. No attempt is made to include all symptoms, but rather to highlight those which particularly involve rehabilitation staff.

ACUTE CONFUSIONAL STATE

This can arise as a result of any acute physical illness, but is reversible if the underlying cause is treated. It can be precipitated by toxins produced by certain drugs or by chest infections, or can follow sudden changes in the normal pattern of life, such as the death of a relative or friend, or a move of home. Patients with an acute confusional state can reach such a level of distress and excitability that any therapeutic intervention is impossible; any active therapy required has to wait until the confusional state has cleared.

DEPRESSION

Depression is one of the most common mental disorders of older people, occurring more often in women than men. This disorder, characterized by abnormally lowered mood, may develop over a period of weeks or months. Patients show a loss of interest in life and neglect their personal hygiene and appearance. They find it difficult if not impossible to make decisions and carry out essential daily activities; they may feel frustrated as a result and treat those around them with aggression and hostility. Sleep and appetite are frequently disturbed, with a consequent loss of weight and lack of energy. Intelligence is not affected, although poor concentration and memory may give the impression that it is. The risk of suicide or the inability to cope with everyday life often necessitates admission to hospital.

During the treatment period in hospital, anti-depressant drugs are prescribed. In some cases if the condition does not respond to drug therapy or if the depression is particularly severe, electroconvulsive therapy (ECT) may be given. This physical treatment remains controversial, but can provide an effective and rapidly acting treatment when applied to carefully selected patients (Brandon *et al.*, 1984). Rehabilitation staff are likely to be involved in treating patients' mental and physical problems.

PARAPHRENIA

A less common mental illness, paraphrenia tends to affect women more than men. It is thought to be a form of schizophrenia arising for the first time in those who are over the age of 60 years. The main symptoms are paranoid delusions, with the false ideas so firmly fixed that no amount of reasoning can alter them. The anxiety associated with the delusions may necessitate referral for therapy.

DEMENTIA

The term dementia is used for a cluster of signs and symptoms characterized by a generalized and irremediable impairment of intellect, memory and personality. The decline is progressive and permanent. Dementia of the Alzheimer type (DAT) mainly affects women and results in a steady decline in ability, whereas multi-infarct dementia (MID) is more likely to affect men. In MID there is a characteristic step-wise deterioration due to a series of mini-strokes. Other early-onset dementias occurring before the age of 65 include Huntington's chorea and the much rarer Pick's and Creuzfeldt–Jakob diseases.

It is now thought that DAT is made up of several different neuro-pathologies which are gradually being identified, Lewy body cortical disease (LBCD) being one of them. They all show the characteristics of DAT as well as those associated with the other neuropathology.

People with dementia often pose many difficult management problems and have profound personality changes. Short-term memory is commonly affected in varying degrees of severity and patients become increasingly disorientated in time, place and person. Long-term memory remains remarkably intact until the later stages of the disease. If patients retain enough insight and are aware of these deficiencies, depression may well accompany the dementia. Communicating with patients becomes a major problem, since there may be expressive as well as receptive dysphasic-type problems. Misinterpretation of other people's actions or intentions can result in unexpected outbursts of aggression, whilst the inability to interpret the surroundings may provoke anxiety and fear. Mobility problems may develop as the dementia progresses, affecting walking and general functioning. Balance is often impaired, and falls become frequent occurrences. Self-care skills also decrease, until bathing, dressing, toileting and finally feeding need full assistance. There is virtually a reversal of the development stages of a child.

ASSESSMENT

MENTAL STATUS TESTS AND RATING SCALES

It is possible to measure the extent of the patients' problems, since mental status tests are available for this purpose; there are many different types. Clinical psychologists or doctors usually carry out the more intricate and time consuming tests but nursing staff or other personnel may complete shorter ones. Occupational therapists and speech and language therapists can contribute to the diagnostic procedure.

Mental status tests are carried out for a specific purpose. For example, information about patients' mental state can be obtained from the Mini Mental State Examination (Folstein, Folstein and McHugh, 1974) and cognitive function can be tested by the Kendrick Battery (Gibson and Kendrick, 1979). Other tests measure behaviour and the severity of the depressed state.

It is not appropriate to describe these tests in detail. However, an example of a simple memory test (Table 8.1) is included; this can be carried out quickly by a key worker or designated team member as part of their assessment procedure.

Table 8.1 Twelve questions which form the information/orientation sub-test of the Cognitive Assessment Scale taken from the Clifton Assessment Procedure for the Elderly (Pattie and Gilleard, 1979)

 1. What's your name?
 2. How old are you?
 3. What is your date of birth?
 4. What is this place/Where are you now?
 5. What is your home address?
 6. What is the name of this town/city?
 7. Who is the Prime Minister?
 8. Who is the President of the United States of America?
 9. What are the colours of the British flag/Union Jack?
10. What day is it? (NB Not date)
11. What month is it?
12. What year is it?

The number of correct answers are scored out of the possible 12. Patients with depression are expected to score 8 or more, whilst those with dementia are likely to achieve 7 or less.

FUNCTIONAL RATING SCALES

There are many different scales which measure function (see Chapter 7), including the hierarchically based Index of Independence of ADL (Katz and Akpom, 1976), the Barthel index (Granger, Albrecht and Hamilton, 1979) and the Functional Independence Measure (State University of New York, 1990); any of these could be used with older people suffering from depression. The ADL-Oriented Assessment of Mobility (Pomeroy, 1990) has been developed specifically for use with patients with dementia. As described in Chapter 7, the advantage and disadvantage of each must be considered.

FUNCTIONAL ABILITY

Test results, medical history and assessment findings of individual team members enable staff to gain a good general impression of the patients' mental state and a relatively clear idea of what they might be able and need to achieve mentally and physically. Further information is obtained from carers, formal and informal. These comprehensive data create a baseline from which personalized goals can be jointly agreed, and changes in ability can be measured (see also Chapter 7).

The patients' response to group activities and from activities of daily living (ADL) help to determine which areas of ADL need particular consideration. These may include reading, listening to the radio, watching television, writing, going out and hobbies. Functional activities may include shopping, cooking, cleaning, laundry, mobility (transfers, walking, stairs, moving on and off the bed), bathing, dressing, eating and drinking.

THE MENTAL AND PHYSICAL LINK

There is a demonstrable link between poor physical performance and mental state in older people with mental illness. In depression and dementia, functional mobility and independence in ADL may be severely affected, but as a result of quite different mechanisms, which will be described later. To further complicate the picture, multiple pathology is common in old age; joint stiffness, muscle weakness, sensory loss, the effects of drugs and limited exercise tolerance, for example, additionally influence the level of the patients' performance and affect their mood. Social factors such as poor housing, poverty, isolation and bereavement can also make an immense impact on the physical and mental health of older people.

PARTICULAR POINTS TO CONSIDER DURING ASSESSMENT

The establishment of CMHTs has enabled many more assessments to be carried out in the community than in the past. The most appropriate assessment is the one that is carried out in the patients' home. Surrounded by familiar possessions, using well known equipment and following their usual routine, patients demonstrate a much more reliable result. An assessment carried out in the hospital can only reflect the patients' performance at that time and in that place. The assessment is carried out on the lines described in Chapter 7. There are, however, particular points that need to be emphasized during the assessment:

* the assessment is carried out in a courteous manner;
* the time of day is appropriate;
* the assessment finishes on a positive note.

DEPRESSED PATIENTS

Depressed patients may show a great lack of interest and concentration and give the erroneous impression that they do not understand what is being asked of them. Staff need to remind themselves that the patients' intellect is not affected, even if memory is temporarily impaired. A low-key approach is required and the assessor must give patients time to express themselves and be ready to listen patiently to what they are saying. The reasons for the assessment are always clearly explained to patients, who may need to be gently persuaded to co-operate.

The patients' mood may well vary from day to day; therefore, if they are obviously having an 'off day', it is best not to proceed with the assessment and, in spite of service pressures, to return at another time.

PATIENTS WITH DEMENTIA

People with dementia frequently have difficulty in locating the source of sound or speech, but addressing them by name minimizes the problem. Very clear and concise explanations and requests are always given so that patients have the best opportunity of understanding. In some cases, assessors may judge that patients are unlikely to understand, but should nevertheless give them the benefit of the doubt and address them as if they do; those with dementia have the same rights as any other older people (King's Fund Centre, 1986) (see also Chapter 4).

Non-verbal communication is particularly effective with people with dementia, so the use of a friendly facial expression, a non-threatening body posture and position, and the caring, reassuring use of touch should be exploited. It is unwise to talk about patients suffering from mental illness within their hearing or to appear to be discussing them from a distance.

Following admission to hospital or a move to unfamiliar surroundings within the community, patients may require several days to settle down before assessment is attempted. The psychological impact of a move could adversely affect the results of an assessment carried out too soon, although pressure for faster throughput may compromise these best intentions. Patients with MID can be expected to show partic ularly well defined variations in mood and physical performance from hour to hour as well as from day to day.

The results of more than one assessment of ADL or functional ability are required, in order for a realistic report to be prepared. The report should clearly indicate the range of assistance required for each task, so that misunderstandings do not occur. There is a considerable difference between 'significant physical help' and 'verbal guidance'. In both cases one person is occupied with the patient for approximately the same length of time, but a physically strong carer is needed for the former.

IDENTIFICATION OF PROBLEMS

A problem list is drawn up at the conclusion of assessments carried out by individual team members. This is likely to include problems of a medical, psychiatric, social, behavioural, physical and functional nature. It is, however, advisable to note patients' strengths as well as weaknesses. Some problems can be avoided or lessened; for example, physical performance can be increased if any sensory deficits are minimized simply by ensuring that any prescribed spectacles, footwear, walking aids, hearing aids, dentures, etc. are available if normally used (see Chapters 11 and 15). Depersonalization in hospital or nursing/ residential home can be decreased if patients have a few possessions of their own around them and wear their own clothes.

SEATING

The importance of appropriate seating cannot be overstated. Occupational therapists or physiotherapists should be able to offer sound advice on solving or easing patients' seating problems (Institute for Consumer Ergonomics, 1983). Seating can have a profound effect upon mobility. For example, a seat height which is appropriate to stature can facilitate performance, whereas an unusually low one can imprison. Special chairs that have an exaggerated seat rake (up to 25°) can have a similar effect. Since the patients' hips are at a considerably lower level than their knees, rising is made more difficult or impossible. The deliberate and protracted use of such chairs, to restrict the activity of restless mobile patients, can ultimately render them immobile, as there is a high risk of the development of hip and knee contractures. However, used appropriately, special chairs can be both effective and comfortable and solve many problems. It is good practice for special chairs to be used as part of a comprehensive treatment plan at the recommendation of an occupational therapist or physiotherapist who has assessed the patient's needs.

GOAL SETTING

Following the drawing up of the problem list, goals are agreed and set. This process should involve the patient, although in most cases a close relative or home carer needs to be included as well. This is particularly important when patients are suffering from dementia, but they should be given every opportunity to contribute.

There are many other problems specific either to depression or to dementia which require treatment or management. These will be considered separately and details of the intervention will be given. The role of occupational therapy and physiotherapy in psychiatry is comprehensively discussed by Findlay (1988) and Everett, Dennis and Ricketts (1995).

MANAGEMENT OF PROBLEMS ASSOCIATED WITH DEPRESSION

Patients with moderate depression are treated at home, but may be offered group therapy at their local mental health centre. Those who are severely ill need to be admitted into hospital for intensive care; the severity of the depression and the increasing inability to cope with the demands of everyday life necessitate this. Admission is also precipitated if there is a real risk of suicide. Therapy is directed towards the patients' state of mind and to their intellectual, social and functional problems, whether they are at home or in hospital. In order to promote 'ownership' and maximum co-operation, the plan of treatment should be discussed with and agreed by the patient whenever possible. It should be realistic and achievable.

The patients' self esteem is probably low and they may lack confidence and motivation. They are therefore encouraged to participate in activities that can be easily achieved. Initially, simple everyday house-keeping tasks, such as washing and drying dishes, may be indicated, in order to improve their morale through contribution. The level of difficulty of the activity chosen depends very much on the severity of the depression, with the more complex tasks being introduced as the patients' condition improves. There may be feelings of guilt and un-worthiness, in which case individual counselling sessions may be appropriate. Any suicidal threats voiced during therapy should always be taken seriously and reported immediately to nursing or medical staff.

GROUP WORK

Participation in groups gives patients an opportunity to practise other skills. Quizzes, drama or other activity groups encourage them to communicate and exercise intellectual abilities as well as improving social interaction. Relaxation training may be given for the anxiety which often accompanies depression. There are many different methods of relaxation, including autogenics (Schultz and Luthe, 1959), progressive relaxation (Jacobsen, 1965) and the Mitchell method of physiological relaxation (Mitchell, 1977). Scripts for the above and details of other techniques are given by Heptenstall (1995) in a chapter on relaxation training (see also Chapter 7).

Complementary therapies continue to be popular with patients (Dennis *et al.*, 1995). Therapists who have undertaken additional training courses, and have the necessary professional indemnity cover, are using, where appropriate, acupuncture/acupressure, aromatherapy, reflex-therapy/reflexology as part of the patients' therapy. Physiotherapists are also making more use of their traditional massage skills than in the recent past.

HOSTILITY, AGGRESSION AND LACK OF CO-OPERATION

Depressed patients often express intense anger and hostility towards those around them (Weissman, Klerman and Paykel, 1971). This stems from frustration caused by their inability to function as before and because of difficulties in communicating their real fears and worries.

They may initially be uncooperative when asked to help on the ward or attend a therapy session, not caring to face the fact that they are unable to carry out everyday tasks without assistance, or fearing failure in public. If this occurs, it is advisable to wait a couple of days before try-ing again. Then gentle coaxing may persuade them to participate in an activity such as a simple woodwork session, perhaps on an individual basis at first, where there is an end product. They are then able to boost their self esteem by giving the item to relatives or other patients. Positive feedback in the form of praise enhances the likelihood of further co-operation. Other activities can then be introduced, beginning with the ones which patients are known to enjoy. Gardening is often a favourite.

Patients may often show hostility or aggression towards staff or other patients who try too hard to persuade them to join in. It may be decided that for such patients it is more appropriate for them to sit and watch a group activity taking place. It is possible that at a later date their inter-est will be stimulated enough for them to find the confidence to join in. These same patients may later feel guilty about their aggressive behaviour and need to be reassured that no offence was caused by it.

Disappointment can also cause aggression. This can best be avoided by always suggesting tasks that are well within patients' physical and mental capabilities. Depressed patients feel vulnerable and need plenty of sympathetic care. As the depression responds to treatment and the patient's condition improves, any inappropriate behaviour usually ceases.

A small proportion of patients develop very severe physical problems and become virtually immobile. There is often an underlying physical condition such as osteoarthritis which is causing pain and stiffness.

These patients may complain of symptoms which they would normally tolerate well (Grimley Evans, 1986). Reassurances are needed in the form of explanations about the effect of depression on their tolerance of pain. Some local physiotherapy may be given to help relieve the pain; it is usually most effective if carried out in conjunction with active functional rehabilitation. Advice on positioning and appropriate seating is important to avoid poor sitting posture and to enable patients to rise from sitting as easily as possible. General exercise group sessions, with or without music, also make a valuable contribution and add variety to the programme. The skills of a music therapist may be available in some services.

Elderly depressed patients are particularly susceptible to infections. This is due to the general loss of motivation associated with the depression which results in a dramatic decrease in their normal level of physical activity. An acute chest infection can have a systemic effect and quickly cause immobility. A concerted team effort is needed to ensure that pressure sores (Norton, McLaren and Exton-Smith, 1962) or soft-tissue contractures are not allowed to develop during this period. It is essential that a programme of frequent and regular changes of position, making use of a comfortable chair as well as the bed, is agreed and supervised, in order to avoid these problems. Pressure relieving cushions, mattresses and other approaches should be used immediately. Patients should also be assisted to achieve a good stretch in the standing position during weight-bearing transfers from bed to chair or commode, in order to prevent soft-tissue contractures.

RETURNING HOME

When patients are considered well enough physically and mentally, preparations are made for the return home. An occupational therapist or nurse may accompany them on several home visits in order to ascertain whether they are able to complete essential household tasks safely in familiar surroundings. This is of particular importance if patients are returning to live alone. It may of course be necessary for therapy to be continued on an out-patient basis at the day hospital.

MANAGEMENT OF PROBLEMS ASSOCIATED WITH DEMENTIA

Much of the therapy is nowadays carried out in the community, the patients' own home, the residential/nursing home or the day hospital. The problems associated with dementia need to be managed during therapy; the assessment highlights those which require particular attention. The overall aim is to enable patients to be as independent as possible and to ease the carers' task. If mobility problems are particularly severe, carers may need to be encouraged to use some mechanical aids to ease heavy handling. Rehabilitation staff should therefore be well informed about aids and equipment that are available and proficient in training others in their use.

COMMUNICATION

Difficulties in communication are often a major problem, even with the use of all the necessary aids required for enhancing vision, hearing and speech. In order to get the message across to patients it may be necessary to use written as well as verbal and non-verbal methods. Progress may depend a great deal on effective communication. The patients' difficulty in understanding may be further increased by poor concentration; it is therefore often possible to engage in only short bursts of activity or participation interspersed with rests or pauses. Communication is a two-way process, so it is equally important to listen carefully to what patients say and to make determined efforts to understand what they mean. General approaches to communication are described in Chapter 9. Some additional ways of communicating with dementia patients are now suggested.

Giving instructions

Patients need time to understand, so well spaced repetition of instructions is essential. Care is, however, needed with the instruction itself. A 'direct' request such as 'Stand up, please' is preferable to 'Would you like to stand up?' The latter 'indirect' question form invites the possibility of a 'No' response and is therefore best avoided!

Negatively expressed instruction may lead to patients carrying out the opposite and undesired action. For example, a warning 'Don't sit down' given to a patient who is threatening to sit on an imaginary chair may encourage him to do just that, since he appears not to hear the negative. A positively phrased instruction such as 'Stand up' or 'Stay standing' is more likely to be effective.

Phraseology used locally may be more readily understood by older patients than the words or expressions normally used by staff who do not come from the locality. Experimentation with wording or words is worthwhile and can be rewarding. Communication with patients from different cultures requires a similarly explorative approach (see Chapter 3).

The careful wording of a single instruction to cover a sequence of movements can often successfully elicit a response at subcortical level, where a series of instructions for the same sequence of movements may fail when patients try to organize their response at a conscious level. For example, 'Come and help me lay the table' encompasses the unstated tasks of standing up and walking across the room for the given purpose of laying the table. This strategy enables patients who have difficulty in the conscious organization of some movements to do them automatically whilst distracted by a request to carry out another task.

Using cues

Communication can be enhanced by using cues. For example, a touch cue applied with a slight upward and forward pressure on the upper back of an appropriately positioned patient supplements the verbal request; a gentle tapping of the hips of a patient carrying out chair-to-chair transfers helps to indicate the direction of the turn required; and a sound cue made by smacking the seat of a chair attracts the patient's attention and adds to his/her understanding of the spoken request to 'Sit here, please'. Many different cues can be devised to encourage the required movement or activity.

DISORIENTATION

Orientation problems cause distress to patients with dementia and particularly to those who have some insight remaining. Reminiscence therapy, which makes use of the patients' more intact long-term memory, may help to bring them up to date with the present. Cards (see Useful addresses) make excellent visual aids for this purpose and enable conversation to take place on such varied subjects as transport, shopping and weddings. Comparisons between past memories and the present reality are emphasized.

Reality orientation (Rimmer, 1982) is directed more towards patients' short-term memory problems. When it is used in the 24-h format by everyone in contact with patients, constant reminders help to keep them in touch with what is going on around them. The techniques can be used by carers at home as well as by hospital personnel. When the patients' ability to converse is strictly limited, it is useful for carers who are physically assisting them to give a running commentary on each action being carried out. This provides a meaningful substitute for one-sided social chatting.

It is particularly important that the structure and order of a normal day are maintained, since night and day reversal can occur. It is therefore desirable to have a large clock with a traditional face positioned where it can be easily seen; a digital clock is unfamiliar to older people and therefore unacceptable. If patients are being cared for at home, it may be helpful to have a notice on the wall giving their name and address. In a hospital or a residential/nursing home setting a reality orientation board showing various details such as the name of the place and the day and date are often provided – but they do need to be correct to prevent disorientation of patients – and staff!

MEMORY PROBLEMS

Undue memory loss makes it increasingly difficult for patients to carry out ADL in the correct sequence. Cues can once again help to minimize the problem. For example, the occupational therapist re-training patients to dress themselves arranges the clothes in a logical and familiar order, so that cues to the sequence are provided. Carers are also encouraged to use the same method each time patients dress. The importance of reinforcing a particular pattern with frequent and identical repetition cannot be over-stressed. It is possible that patients may forget what they are doing in mid-activity, so they should be given the necessary prompts to help them accomplish the task in hand.

AGGRESSION

Patients with dementia often show aggression and hostility to those around them. They may use verbal abuse in the form of shouting or swearing or show physical aggression by hitting out, kicking or spitting. There are some situations which render this type of behaviour more likely, for example the increased disorientation experienced in strange surroundings; the state of anxiety induced by the late arrival of a meal or visitor; and any unexpected demands made on unprepared patients. Frequent explanations and reminders are needed to reassure and prepare patients, so that aggressive responses are avoided. The stability of a well structured day, such as that in an institutional setting, often seems to suit the needs of these patients. Home carers should be made aware of the benefits engendered by a stable routine.

The cause of the aggression is not always apparent, so staff may wish to investigate occurrences which immediately preceded the inappropriate behaviour. If trigger factors are identified, they should be shared by all staff, and avoided. Better behaviour can be reinforced by spending time with patients when they are not aggressive. The ABC of behavioural analysis (Stokes, 1990) offers a structured approach which enables professional carers to understand better the reasons for patients' challenging behaviour and to seek possible solutions.

Physically active dementia patients, who like to wander at will, often become restless and aggressive if space is limited and there is no access to an enclosed garden. Goodwin (1984) has suggested that 'wanderers' are those who stroll further than is comfortable to whoever is in charge! In the hospital setting the necessary freedom of movement can be achieved by taking such patients for a long walk in the corridors or, if the weather allows, in the grounds. In the domestic or residential home setting, walking inside may not be an option, so walks in the neighbourhood or trips to the local shops may be the only possibilities. The internal design of a modern nursing home catering for people with dementia should be such that corridors provide for the needs of wanderers during inclement weather and give access to an enclosed garden space.

Anxiety and aggression can be avoided during therapy by giving patients time to carry out the required activities at their own pace. Dysphasic patients may become frustrated by their inability to communicate and respond by lashing out. (Guidelines for dealing with dysphasia are covered in Chapter 9.)

PAIN AND FEAR

Patients who have fallen several times while walking may understandably become afraid of doing so when they move. They may as a result refuse or be reluctant to leave the safe haven of their chair. Dragging them out will only increase their anxiety and resistance. The traditional placing of a walking aid in front of the patient may provide sufficient reassurance to some, whilst others may initially require a more familiar and solid looking form of support, such as the back of a readily available dining chair. The chair fills the space in front of the patient and offers solid visual reassurance. It is important that patients are encouraged to *push down with both hands on the arms of their own chair* to assist themselves to rise before holding onto the support, so that a safe pattern becomes automatic.

Patients may also show great fear when being moved on the bed. Reassurance and slow careful physical handling can minimize this fear by giving them time to adjust to any changes in position. Whilst being assisted to rise from the bed to sit on the edge, the sight of the drop to the floor may alarm the patient. The view of the floor can be temporarily blocked by the assistant positioning him/herself close to the bed and level with the patient's head. Similarly, the patient's fear of descending the stairs can be minimized if the assistant steps down first, facing the patient and therefore partly blocking the alarming void ahead and at the same time observing their reactions.

All those involved in patients' care should be made aware of the strategies that have been recommended by different disciplines to minimize difficulties, so that they can be used consistently.

Physiotherapists are often faced with the necessity of carrying out movements which can cause pain. Following a recently repaired hip fracture, surrounding muscles may be sensitive and pain-killing drugs are usually necessary before treatment. The progression of treatment following fractures often has to be unusually slow until the pain subsides. An empathic approach to patients' fears and anxieties helps to minimize much of the aggression which might otherwise occur during rehabilitation.

MISINTERPRETING THE ENVIRONMENT

Patients with dementia are affected by their surroundings and often have great difficulty in making sense of them. Their impaired ability to interpret what they see may well be exacerbated by poor eyesight. Jazzy patterns on a carpet may be taken for objects spilt on the floor and patients may try to pick them up. A self-reflection in a mirror or window may be interpreted as an intruder and can cause great distress. A shaft of sunlight shining on the floor can bring patients to a stop or cause them to walk over or round it. They may step very deliberately up and over a silver-coloured threshold strip or a long dark area of pattern on the flooring, interpreted as a step, landing heavily as a result of the misjudged action. This 'stepping response' may upset balance and cause a fall. When assisting patients who show such a response, firm and repeated reassurances should be given that the floor is flat. Carers should be encouraged to reassure patients in similar situations, acting as 'interpreter' of the surroundings on their behalf. Planning accommodation and furnishings for such patients requires considerable practical experience.

MOBILITY PROBLEMS

Staff must manage the problems associated with dementia whilst attempting to promote some useful functional mobility (Oddy, 1987). Strategies for minimizing these were suggested earlier. Key issues for people with dementia with mobility problems are therefore:

- explorative approach to communication
- use of cues
- strategies to boost confidence
- short episodes of activity
- suitable furniture and aids.

Individual sessions are essential for specific re-training, but group exercises with small pieces of brightly coloured apparatus offer valuable opportunities for additional stimulation. With patients seated on dining-type chairs, group exercises provide variety and contribute positively to the patients' mental, physical and social well being. Exercises with a colourful 'parachute' are also popular; this piece of apparatus can be used with the patients seated or standing in a circle. Each grasps the edge in front of them and rhythmically raises and lowers the canopy exercising balance, limbs, and co-ordination. Gratifying and unexpected results are often obtained spontaneously during an enjoyable group exercise session – especially when music is used.

PROBLEMS WITH ADL

The importance of maintaining the normal order and structure of the day as far as possible has already been stated. The need to practise tasks at the relevant time of day has also been discussed. Patients are much more likely to complete a task successfully when using familiar equipment, with traditional methods in familiar surroundings.

RE-TRAINING ADL

If patients are unable to carry out tasks unaided, verbal prompting or assistance is given to ensure their smooth completion. It may be necessary for the sequence to be demonstrated carefully, as for example during meal preparation, and for other tasks, such as shaving or teeth-cleaning, to be carried out on the patient themselves. Repetition and regular practice facilitate the re-learning of tasks if they are within the patients' capability.

Domestic and household chores, together with self-care activities, are complex in nature and consist of skills that have been learnt and perfected over many years. Most of these activities involve the necessity to carry out each stage in a particular order, something which patients with dementia find increasingly difficult. The decline in intellectual processes and memory gradually tend to deprive patients of their ability to care for themselves.

MINIMIZING PROBLEMS

There are many simple ways of minimizing patients' difficulties by making use of:

- appropriate aids and equipment
- cues.

Aids and equipment

Feeding aids can be very effective: a non-slip Dycem mat prevents plates from travelling across the table, a plate guard helps to keep food on the plate and a non-spill feeder can be managed by patients when the use of a cup becomes impracticable. All should be supplied as a result of a personalized assessment and not provided universally, irrespective of need.

Showering can replace bathing, either when patients are no longer able to retain their balance, or when handling problems are being experienced by carers. Hand-held showers are usually preferred to an overhead type.

Selecting clothing with manageable fastenings can facilitate the ability to dress independently. An occupational therapist can provide guidance on clothing and Disabled Living Centres are also a source of help.

Cues

The complicated process of making a cup of tea or dressing can be eased if the items to be used are laid out in a logical order beforehand.

ENCOURAGING ACTIVITY AT HOME

Patients with dementia who are being maintained at home may need a great deal of support. Input from a home care worker or home help may be available, but regular monitoring should be provided by the community psychiatric nurse, social worker or therapist and co-operation of the relatives and willing neighbours encouraged.

The patient may not be able to carry out normal complex household and domestic chores, but should be encouraged to remain active in the home. There are some easy tasks which elderly female patients enjoy doing, probably badly, but nevertheless they purposefully occupy time. Such tasks consist of dusting, sweeping, arranging flowers and washing small amounts of clothes. Elderly male patients often enjoy pottering in the garden. It will be interesting to note if future 'liberated' generations return to traditional gender responsibility tasks when mental illness dulls fashionable choice. The occupational therapist can advise carers on which ADL tasks the patient can reasonably and safely be expected to do.

Physiotherapists should also liaise closely with those who are caring for patients and make sure that they are aware of any changes in their capabilities as re-training progresses. Carers need to be competent and willing. They need to prove themselves able to carry out the routine practice delegated to them. These delegated activities should be such that they are easily incorporated into the patients' day. Since they are likely to consist of practising rising to standing, transfers and walking, they should be achievable. They should be carried out frequently and in the manner recommended by the physiotherapist. It is not reasonable to expect relatives or home carers who are already under considerable pressure to carry out any additional practice of a more complex nature.

PREDICTING THE OUTCOME OF REHABILITATION

DEPRESSION

The eventual outcome for severely depressed patients with mobility and self-care problems is generally good. The period of time involved may be long and is linked to the lifting of the depression. Patients' physical performance and mental state should be expected eventually to return near to that which existed prior to the depressive illness.

DEMENTIA

Even a minor illness such as a common cold may be enough to upset the fragile balance between ability and inability and cause patients with dementia to go 'off their feet'. This does not necessarily mean that their walking days are over. Even after a bout of bronchopneumonia, the previous level of mobility can often be re-established with an encouraging approach and a very gradual re-introduction of functional activities and walking. A similarly positive attitude can be adopted towards the recovery expected following fractures and small strokes, although each incident must inevitably result in some loss of ability, irrespective of the dementia.

In spite of the progressive nature of dementia and the fact that it is not curable, much can be done to ease the patients' problems and those of their carers, and perhaps slow the deterioration. Therapy may consist of a daily concentrated session, but the outcome may depend upon how much additional practice can be incorporated into the rest of the day by carers or other members of the team. This applies whether patients are at home or in hospital. When the agreed goals have been achieved and reassessment indicates that the optimum progress has been made, the maintenance task passes to family or other carers who are supporting the patient on a daily basis. It is advisable to offer open access for advice and possible reassessment to these carers.

SUMMARY

The mental state and physical function of elderly people are very much interlinked. An examination of the problems associated with depression or dementia highlights this situation. However, the content and scope of the programme of activities selected for patients with depression are very different from those required by patients with dementia. Clinically depressed patients are expected to make a good recovery; the low mood gradually lifts with treatment and normal function is usually restored. Patients with dementia do not recover; intellectual capability slowly declines and physical functioning deteriorates. However, the maintenance of some aspects of mobility for as long as possible helps them to retain a degree of independence and to delay the onset of the physical and psychological suffering associated with immobility. Assessment and treatment planning must therefore be personalized, implemented faithfully by all team members and regularly reviewed.

All team members have a significant role to play in the multidisciplinary team involved in the mental and physical care of these elderly patients and in the support of their carers; any of them may well be key workers.

REFERENCES

Age Concern (undated) *Abuse of Elderly People – Guidelines for Action*, Age Concern, London.

Brandon, S., Cowley, P., McDonald, C., Neville, P., Palmer, R. and Wellstood-Eason, S. (1984) Electroconvulsive therapy: results in depressive illness from the Leicestershire trial. *British Medical Journal*, **288**, 22–5.

Dennis, M., Dunham, L., Jones, C. and Holey, E. (1995) Complementary medicine, in *Physiotherapy in Mental Health*, (eds T. Everett, M. Dennis and E. Ricketts), Butterworth Heinemann, Oxford, pp. 252–80.

Everett, T., Dennis, M. and Ricketts, E. (eds) (1995) *Physiotherapy in Mental Health*, Butterworth Heinemann, Oxford.

Findlay, L. (1988) *Occupational Therapy Practice in Psychiatry*, Chapman & Hall, London.

Folstein, M.F., Folstein, S.E. and McHugh, P.R. (1974) Mini Mental State: a practical method for grading the cognitive state of patients for the clinician. *Journal of Psychiatric Research*, **12**(3), 189–98.

Gibson, A.J. and Kendrick, D.C. (1979) *The Kendrick Battery for the Detection of Dementia in the Elderly*, NFER Publishing, Windsor, Ontario.

Goodwin, S. (1984) On desolation row. *New Age*, **Autumn**, 22–7.

Granger, C.V., Albrecht, G.L. and Hamilton, B.B. (1979) Outcome of comprehensive medical rehabilitation; measurement by PULSES profile and the Barthel index. *Archives of Physical Medical Rehabilitation*, **60**, 145–54.

Grimley Evans, J. (1986) The interaction between physical and psychiatric disease in the elderly. *Update*, **February**, 265–70.

Heptenstall, S.T. (1995) Relaxation training, in *Physiotherapy in Mental Health*, Butterworth Heinemann, Oxford, pp. 188–208.

Institute for Consumer Ergonomics (1983) *Selecting Easy Chairs for Elderly and Disabled People*, University of Technology, Loughborough.

Jacobsen, E. (1965) *Progressive Relaxation*, 2nd edn, University of Chicago Press, Chicago.

Katz, S. and Akpom, C.A. (1976) A measure of primary sociobiological function. *International Journal of Health Services*, **6**(3), 493–508.

Kay, D.W.K., Beamish, P. and Roth, M. (1964) Old age mental disorders in Newcastle upon Tyne. *British Journal of Psychiatry*, **110**, 146–58.

King's Fund Centre (1986) *Living Well into Old Age*, King's Fund Centre, London.

Kingston, P. and Phillipson, C. (1994) Elder abuse and neglect. *British Journal of Nursing*, 3(22), 1171–90.

Lindesay, J., Briggs, K. and Murphy, E. (1989) The Guy's/Age Concern Survey: prevalence rates of cognitive impairment, depression and anxiety in an urban elderly community. *British Journal of Psychiatry*, **155**, 317–29.

Lodge, B. (1981) *Coping with Caring*, MIND, London.

Mitchell, L, (1977) *Simple Relaxation*, Murray, London.

North, C., Ritchie, J. and Ward, K. (1993) *Factors Influencing the Implementation of the Care Programme Approach*, HMSO, London.

Norton, D., McLaren, R. and Exton-Smith, A. (1962) Pressure sores, in *Investigations into Geriatric Nursing Problems*, National Corporation for the Care of Old People, London, pp. 193–238, reprinted (1976) by Churchill Livingstone.

Oddy, R.J. (1987) Promoting mobility in patients with dementia: some suggested strategies for physiotherapists. *Physiotherapy Practice*, **1**, 18–28.

Pattie, A.H. and Gilleard, C.J. (1979) *Manual of the Clifton Assessment Procedures for the Elderly (CAPE)*, Hodder and Stoughton Educational, Sevenoaks.

Pomeroy, V. (1990) Development of an ADL oriented assessment-of-mobility scale suitable for use with elderly people with dementia. *Physiotherapy*, 76(8), 446–8.

Rimmer, L. (1982) *Reality Orientation; Principles and Practice*, Winslow Press, Bicester.

Roth, M. (1955) The natural history of mental disorder in old age. *Journal of Mental Science*, **101**, 281–301.

Schultz, J.H. and Luthe, W. (1959) *Autogenic Training: a Psychological Approach to Psychotherapy*, Grune and Stratton, New York and London.

State University of New York (1990) *Guide for the Use of the Uniform Data Set for Medical Rehabilitation Including the Functional Independence Measure (FIM)*, Department of Rehabilitation Medicine, State University of New York, Buffalo.

Stokes, G. (1990) Behavioural analysis, in *Working with Dementia* (eds G. Stokes and F. Goudie), Winslow Press, Bicester.

Weissman, M.M., Klerman, G.L. and Paykel, E.S. (1971) Clinical evaluation of hostility in depression, in *Abnormal Psychology*, 4th edn (eds G.C. Davison and J.M. Neale), Wiley, New York.

FURTHER READING

Alzheimer's Disease Society (1984) *Caring for the Person with Dementia – a Guide for Families and other Carers*, Alzheimer's Disease Society, London.

Kitwood, T. and Bredin, K. (1992) *Person to Person: a Guide to the Care of those with Failing Mental Powers*. Gale Centre Publications, Whitakers Way, Loughton, Essex, IG10 1SQ.

USEFUL ADDRESSES

Winslow Press,
Telford Road,
Bicester,
Oxford OX6 0TS   (for reminiscence cards)

Action on Elder Abuse,
Astral House,
1268 London Road,
London SW16 4ER

Carers National Association,
20–25 Glasshouse Yard,
London EC1A 4JS

Alzheimer's Disease Society,
Gordon House,
10 Green Coat Place,
London SW1 1PA

Institute for Consumer Ergonomics,
University of Technology Loughborough,
75 Swingbridge Road,
Loughborough,
Leicestershire LE11 0JB

Communication problems of older people

9

Kirsten Beining and Jayne Whitaker

NORMAL COMMUNICATION IN OLDER PEOPLE

The term 'communication' encompasses a diverse set of skills which allow human beings to transmit and receive messages. Not only do these skills demand the synergy of voice, speech, language and cognition (Maxim and Bryan, 1994), but they also include the ability to exchange messages through written text and gestural codes.

It is often difficult to separate the traditional linguistic and cognitive skills needed for verbal communication, because demarcation can be misleading and artificial. Voice and speech are produced by transforming respiration into sound and by shaping sounds through articulation to produce speech. Language is the formation of thought into verbal words or written symbols and cognition is the process whereby knowledge is acquired, and includes perception, intuition, memory and reasoning.

The term 'communication' incorporates all these skills with the addition of pragmatics – the use of any of these skills within a particular social context (Davis and Wilcox, 1985). An example of the successful synergy of speech, language, gesture and pragmatics can be observed in everyday communication situations.

Communication skills are affected by the biological ageing process and by pathological changes. It is helpful to differentiate between the two conditions when evaluating the need for intervention. However, despite the need to determine cause and effect, a differential diagnosis is often difficult to make, because of the confounding influences of psychosocial variables such as education, cultural influences, institutionalization and social isolation.

NORMAL COMMUNICATION CHANGES IN OLDER PEOPLE

Biological ageing includes changes to neurocognitive abilities; sensory, motor and musculoskeletal systems, and research indicates the following:

- Verbal and language-mediated tasks do not greatly change with age (Wechsler, 1985; Jarvik, 1962; Cattel, 1963).
- Some aspects of cognition that support language change with increasing age (Rabbitt, 1965; Clarke, 1980).
- Deficits in cognition contribute to the decline in the understanding and use of language (Maccoby, 1971; Rabbitt, 1979).
- Attention deficits may be caused by both visual perceptual and auditory processing abnormalities (Ball *et al.*, 1988; Schonfield, Truman and Kline, 1982).
- The understanding of complex syntax, ambiguous sentences and word or clause order declines with age (Bever, 1970; Maxim, 1982).

LANGUAGE PRODUCTION

Comparative research on language use across the age range has been limited, due to methodological constraints. The important variables of education, cultural differences, dialect and the change in language use and speaking styles have been difficult to control. The increase in performance errors of the older population may be attributed to retrieval difficulties; older subjects need a longer period of time to process and organize language output and fill in this processing time by increasing the frequency of pauses, interjections, sentence repair, etc.

VOICE CHANGES IN SENESCENCE

There are well recognized voice changes during the normal ageing process. Frequency, loudness and rhythm are prone to biological change and have been called senile tremolo. These are due to:

- irregular patterns of expiration during phonation (Luchsinger and Arnold, 1965);
- changes in the respiratory mechanism and endocrine function (Hollien, 1987);
- inappropriate use of a louder voice secondary to impaired hearing which places a strain on the vocal mechanism (see Chapter 15);
- respiratory problems associated with chronic obstructive airway disease, to which the older person is particularly prone;
- changes in natural dentition or badly fitting dentures (see Chapter 15).

Voice change in ageing is most often considered to be secondary to normal biological change. However, the possibility of psychosocial influences such as education, cultural differences and expectations must also be taken into account when establishing why change might have occurred.

COMMUNICATION DISORDERS IN OLDER PEOPLE

The main causes of communication problems in the older patient are:

- stroke
- head injury
- dementia of the Alzheimer type
- multi-infarct dementia
- other degenerative diseases, e.g. Parkinson's disease
- psychiatric conditions, e.g. depression.

In addition to these, a range of social and environmental changes may also affect the ability to communicate. These will be outlined in Associated factors.

Stroke disease is common in older people. The disability that results will depend on the area(s) of cerebral tissue that are affected. Communication disorders that may result, such as aphasia, dysarthria and dyspraxia, are discussed further later.

Traumatic head injury can cause a variety of communication problems, depending on the location of the damage. There is general agreement that individuals who suffer a head injury may exhibit a communication deficit in the form of speech production or language disorder, or both.

Dementia is defined as the global disturbance of higher cortical functions, including memory; the capacity to solve problems of everyday living; the performance of learned perceptuomotor skills; the correct use of social skills and control of emotional reactions, in the absence of clouding of consciousness (Royal College of Physicians Committee on Geriatrics, 1981).

Many of the symptoms of dementia can be mimicked by other conditions; e.g. confusional states and depression can present with similar signs and symptoms. In cortical dementia the effect on communication will usually show a pattern of impairment with more disruption in the use of language than of articulation and grammar.

Language disorders associated with dementia are often referred to as aphasia/dysphasia. Bayles, Tomoeda and Caffrey (1982) identified five differences between communication problems of the aphasic patient, and those of the dementing patient.

1. Aphasia occurs secondary to a sudden onset (e.g. stroke), whereas dementia develops more slowly over time.
2. Deterioration of language in dementia is progressive, but this is not evident in aphasia.
3. Aphasia is due to focal lesions, whereas dementia is accompanied by diffuse brain atrophy.

4. Aphasia has a minimal effect on intellect, whereas loss of reasoning abilities is a primary feature of dementing pathologies.
5. Aphasic patients can present with a dissociation between verbal and non-verbal abilities, whereas most patients with dementia show simultaneous deterioration of both verbal and non-verbal functions.

It is important that these differences are recognized. However, Bayles *et al.* acknowledged that a differential diagnosis often proves difficult, as patients do not always present with discrete signs, but more often with complex communication problems and behaviours which are often seen in both groups, such as fluent aphasia (Gravell, 1988) or progressive dysphasia (Weintraub, Rubin and Marsel-Mesulam, 1990).

Research has shown that subcortical dementia is often associated with dysarthria signs. Speech is characterized by monotony, syllabic stress and fading volume. Often patients do not exhibit language problems which are evident in cortical dementia (Murdoch, 1990).

Multi-infarct dementia (MID), as its name suggests, results from multiple infarctions in the cerebral tissue as a consequence of multiple vessel occlusions (Murdoch, 1990). MID is marked by an abrupt onset with step-wise deterioration and fluctuating progression (Maxim and Bryan, 1994). Signs and symptoms, including speech and language problems, depend on the location of the infarction. According to Bayles, Tomoeda and Caffrey, (1982) the cause is likely to arise from occlusion of the carotid and vertebrobasilar systems.

Parkinson's disease patients are likely to have speech problems in at least 50% of cases (Oxtoby, 1982). Speech is notably dysarthric and some of the main features include breathiness, monotony, altered rate, imprecise articulation and difficulty with initiation (Gravell, 1988). There is also some evidence that language changes occur throughout the duration of the disease (Maxim and Bryan, 1994). It is likely that linguistic behaviour declines in parallel with other cognitive changes (Knight, 1992). Huber, Shuttleworth and Freidenberg (1989) identified difficulties arising from reduced speed in processing information. Other research findings have identified naming difficulties and auditory comprehension difficulties (Matison *et al.* 1982, Lieberman, Friedman and Feldman, 1990).

In **depressive illness** language output can be severely limited, although linguistic competence is not altered (Maxim and Bryan, 1994). Speech and language symptoms include poor attention, lack of interaction, repetition of questions, short phrases and sentences, reduced volume, monotonous intonation, frequent pauses and hesitations. Anecdotal information suggests that a significant proportion of patients attending rehabilitation units suffer from 'low mood' at some point of their treatment. Clinical research indicates that depression is commonly associated as an affective reaction occurring in patients with a speech–language disorder such as aphasia (Wahrborg, 1991). Speech and language therapists may often identify the signs and symptoms of depression in patients who are attending their clinics.

Speech and language therapists working with the older patient are often called on to assist with a differential diagnosis of depression and dementia. They will need to bear in mind the clinical signs and symptoms that are associated with the disorders and liaise with relatives and other healthcare professionals.

TYPES OF COMMUNICATION PROBLEMS

The main types of communication problems are:

- aphasia
- dysarthria
- dyspraxia.

APHASIA

Aphasia is often used interchangeably with dysphasia. The 'a' prefix indicates a total loss of language, and the 'dys' the partial loss of language. The term 'aphasia' in this chapter is defined by The College of Speech and Language Therapists (1991) as follows: 'A language disorder resulting from localized neurological damage. It may present the patient with difficulties in the perception, recognition, comprehension and expression of language through both the verbal and/or written modalities'. There are various types of aphasia.

Non-fluent aphasia

Non-fluent aphasia is associated with a right hemiplegia or hemiparesis. Communication is characterized by the following.

- Understanding is better than expression.
- The patient is aware of his/her errors, is often frustrated and attempts to self correct.
- Spoken output is slow, effortful and telegrammatic, i.e. it consists mainly of content words.
- There are word-finding difficulties.
- There is perseveration.
- The patient is often able to use non-verbal communication such as gesture, pointing and facial expression to convey information.
- The understanding of written material usually mirrors the understanding of spoken language.

- Writing is as commonly impaired as speech, often with misspellings; legibility is often a problem, due to weakness of the hand or the patient having to use the left hand.

Fluent aphasia

This is also known as Wernicke's aphasia and is believed to be caused by a temporoparietal lesion (Murdoch, 1990). Fluent aphasia is not always associated with a hemiplegia or hemiparesis. Communication is characterized by the following.

- Understanding is often severely impaired.
- There are word-finding difficulties – the patient may use non-words in place of real words.
- There is poor awareness of the patient's own errors and few attempts at self correction; consequently the patient is often unaware that a problem exists with communication. A study investigating patients whose fluent aphasia had resolved found that most patients believed that their communication had been either normal or relatively normal (Ross, 1993).
- There is an easy flow of speech, which is often 'empty', lacking in content words and conveying little meaning, though there may be some appropriate language in conjunction with jargon.
- Understanding of written material is also impaired, usually at the same level as the understanding of spoken language, although the visual channel may aid understanding in some patients.
- Writing is abnormal, often resembling the spoken output by lacking meaning.

Global dysphasia presents with a range of accompanying neurological signs representative of severe brain damage. These include visual-field defects, hemiplegia and sensory loss.

Communication is characterized by severe receptive and expressive difficulties. These patients often rely on non-verbal communication, such as gestures and facial expression, to understand spoken language, which is often misinterpreted by relatives and clinicians as an indicator of true understanding of language. If available, expression is often limited to jargon or repetitive stereotyped utterances, which convey little meaning. Reading and writing are equally affected.

DYSARTHRIA

Dysarthria is defined as a 'collective name for a group of related speech disorders that are due to disturbances in muscular control of the speech mechanism resulting from impairment of any of the basic motor processes involved in the execution of speech' (Darley, Aronson and Brown, 1975). Anarthria is the most severe form, with no speech, but vocalizations are still possible.

Traditionally the dysarthrias have been classified in terms of lesion site. However, it may be more helpful to identify the areas of breakdown and undertake a more descriptive analysis of parameters such as respiration, phonation, articulation and resonance, which enables the speech and language therapist to decide upon appropriate management.

DYSPRAXIA

Dyspraxia of speech is defined by Darley, Aronson and Brown (1975) as 'a disorder of motor speech programming manifested primarily by errors in articulation and secondarily by compensatory alterations of prosody. The speaker shows reduced efficiency in accomplishing the oral postures for production of words. The disorder is frequently association with aphasia but may also occur in isolation'.

ASSOCIATED FACTORS INFLUENCING COMMUNICATION

When assessing an older patient's communicative competence it is essential to consider a number of environmental and sensory factors that may have secondary effects on a person's ability to communicate. The following factors will be outlined and discussed:

- environment
- hearing (see also Chapter 15)
- vision and perceptual difficulties (see also Chapter 15).

The environment has a strong influence on communication. 'The improvement of communication skills and opportunities of older individuals in all settings must be considered a right and not a privilege, a priority and not a by-product and a reality not an ideal' (Lubinski, 1981). It is well recognized that a person's ability to communicate is significantly influenced by opportunities to interact, mental and physical stimulation as well as other people with whom he may come into contact. Social isolation is commonplace in the older population, whether the person is still living at home or in residential care. The majority of research has been carried out in settings such as hospitals, nursing homes and rest homes. In many of those settings a 'communication impaired environment' exists (Lubinski, 1984).

The environment can be divided into two sections: the physical and the social environment. The physical environment refers to the layout of furniture (e.g. chairs round the walls which is all too commonplace and often done for the best possible reasons, e.g. safety), lighting, acoustics and privacy. The social environment refers to opportunities to communicate, e.g. discussion groups and communication groups, and not to the TV or radio blaring out pop music or children's programmes. There are many ways to change an environment in order to facilitate communication: indirectly through staff training; altering the physical environment (arranging chairs in groups with good access, so safety is not compromised); and directly through encouraging the setting up of opportunities to interact and communicate, such as giving choices (activities, meals, clothes and outings) and group activities.

In a poor communication environment a communicatively disordered individual's difficulties will often be compounded (Gravell, 1988). As a member of the multidisciplinary team, the speech and language therapist has a major role in advising carers and staff on communication disorders in general and the difficulties of an individual person in particular, in order to ensure awareness of strategies as well as specific activities to facilitate the communication process.

Hearing is dependent on the auditory system, which undergoes a number of changes with age in the outer, middle and particularly the inner ear. Hearing loss is an important factor in communication difficulty for a large number of older people, so it is vital that members of the multidisciplinary team check on hearing abilities of patients and that they are fully aware of the effects of hearing loss on the individual (Maxim and Bryan, 1994). The effects of hearing loss on a person's ability to communicate is well documented in literature (Maxim and Bryan, 1994). There is often a delay before advice is sought which further delays the development of coping strategies (Gravell, 1988). Interaction is often difficult, as obviously the listener role is affected, but the patient's own speech may suffer, e.g. increased loudness. Nonverbal communication is affected, e.g. eye contact is reduced, as the listener concentrates on the speaker's mouth. Helpful strategies include reducing background noise, gaining attention before speaking to the person, facing the person to allow lip-reading and ensuring the light is on the communication partner's face.

Management should include audiological assessment and provision of appropriate amplification aids as well as training in compensatory techniques (Gravell, 1988).

The **visual system** also undergoes changes with ageing. The most common difficulties include cataracts and glaucoma as well as long and short sightedness. Neurological disorders (e.g. stroke) may also cause visual and perceptual difficulties such as neglect, inattention and homonymous hemianopia which need to be considered carefully when assessing a patient. The effects of visual difficulties on communication include direct influences such as reading and writing difficulties, reduced ability in making use of non-verbal communication leading to misunderstandings and indirect influences such as increased isolation.

Helpful strategies include using touch and providing extra information to compensate for loss of non-verbal communication, also taking into account any hearing problems that may be present. Management includes assessment by the appropriate professional and the provision of glasses, magnifying glasses, adapted reading material (e.g. large print) and good lighting (see also Chapter 15).

MANAGEMENT OF COMMUNICATION DIFFICULTIES

Speech and language therapists should become involved at the earliest opportunity, in order to advise on future management. The primary goal of all speech–language therapy intervention for communication disorders is to identify the impairment and to minimize disability and handicap/social disadvantage. The emphasis for management will change as the patient moves through the rehabilitation process. In the acute and early rehabilitation phase the emphasis is on identifying the type of impairment and making predictions about the extent of disability which may occur and what impact this will have on the patient and the family. The ultimate goal in conjunction with the patient/carer is to concentrate on minimizing the impact of social disadvantage that may occur as a result of the original impairment and social isolation. It is generally agreed in the literature that, after assessment, the following treatment/management options should be considered:

- face-to-face therapy
- group therapy
- education and advice to carers
- referral to other agencies.

Initial assessment would attempt to establish a differential diagnosis together with the degree of impairment and handicap (social disadvantage). The speech–language therapist will need to have clear ideas on the following:

- the patient's receptive language skills on formal assessment and in a variety of social situations;
- the patient's motor speech function, i.e. how intelligible they are in a variety of social settings;
- the patient's use (and potential for use) of functional communication strategies, facial expression and augmentative methods of communication to make their needs known;

- the patient's cognitive abilities such as memory and reasoning, and if there are any sensory deficits such as hearing loss, or visual or perceptual disturbances.

Following assessment the therapist will need to discuss future management strategies and options with patients, relatives and other members of the multidisciplinary team. If direct therapy is to be of benefit, a designated block of treatment and goals needs to be agreed between therapist and patient. Communication disorders are often complex and it may be prudent to outline the experimental nature of some forms of intervention, so that therapist, patient and carer do not feel that they have failed if all their goals are not met. Review of goals following a period of treatment is essential in monitoring outcome. It may be that some adjustments will need to be made to goal setting or that an alternative option of management is necessary if primary goals are not being met.

Group therapy has shown positive outcome for patients wishing to improve speech intelligibility (Robertson and Thomson, 1983; Scott and Caird, 1983). This type of approach is also very popular for enhancing total communication strategies in dysphasic patients and helps reduce social isolation. Reminiscence groups also aid social interaction in patients with dementia (see also Chapter 8).

The use of trained assistants to help run groups and to act as a communication facilitator for individual patients is an important resource. In the role of facilitator, such assistants can accompany patients on shopping trips and aid in successful communication exchanges. This type of support can be compared to providing immobile patients with wheelchairs which offers them more access opportunities. By being provided with communication support, i.e. trained assistants, chronic language impaired patients have more opportunities to engage in normal communication events outside the home or care setting.

Education and advice to relatives/carers is essential in ameliorating communication disability. The patient's communication partners need to understand the cause of the difficulty and its manifestations in order to engage in successful communication exchanges and capitalize on the use of compensatory strategies.

The speech–language therapist will need to know how to advise members of the multidisciplinary team on how best to facilitate successful communication between themselves and the language-disordered patient. It is therefore essential that therapists work alongside their colleagues in the therapy, nursing and medical professions to understand their role and in which ways communication can be enhanced. Speech–language therapists should never underestimate the benefits of this reciprocal approach to management and education. Both authors of this chapter have regular opportunities to work in a multidisciplinary team and are aware of the huge benefits to patients, their colleagues and their own knowledge.

The speech–language therapist may need to refer the patient to other agencies such as healthcare professionals or support groups in the voluntary sector such as the Stroke Association, Parkinson's Disease Society, etc.

COMMUNICATION CHARTS

Managing communication disorders in the acute care setting is often a challenging business. Communication charts or aids may be given or requested by colleagues with the best intentions, but patients may be unable to use them for a variety of reasons. Patients' difficulties with using communication charts/aids include:

- diminished consciousness level
- impaired concentration/attention
- visual/perceptual impairment
- inability to recognize symbols, letters or words
- lack of knowledge or practice in using communication charts to indicate their needs or convey information.

Patients need to adjust to the situation and it is often more helpful for those conversing with the patient to use the following strategies:

- watch the patient's face, maintain eye contact where possible, use appropriate facial expression;
- keep sentences short and to the point;
- observe the patient's reaction to gauge if they are listening to you;
- allow pauses of silence while the patient processes what is being said;
- be prepared to repeat, rephrase, demonstrate, write or draw your question if necessary (think what it must be like trying to communicate in a foreign country where nobody understands you. What can you do to get the message across?);
- encourage the patient to respond to you in any way that conveys their meaning;
- use routine situations such as washing and dressing and mealtimes to encourage patients to communicate;
- ask key questions regarding the lavatory, drink, pain, relatives, etc;
- if you completely fail to understand the patient, or they you, admit to the problem and say you will try again later. Do not pretend you have understood the communication attempt if you haven't.

Case history

OM, aged 74, was admitted to a non-acute rehabilitation ward 4 weeks post-onset of stroke from an acute unit. The reasons for transfer were severe communication problems, and non-compliance with rehabilitation goals (at this time awaiting appointment of speech–language therapist in acute unit). The admitting consultant felt that the availability of speech and language therapy was crucial to meeting OM's rehabilitation goals.

Initial assessment showed moderate receptive and severe expressive dysphasia as well as reading and writing difficulties. OM made very good use of facial expression and gesture. The initial goals were as follows:

- encourage use of facial expression and gestures by OM as well as staff and relatives to aid OM's understanding;
- encourage automatic speech, e.g. counting;
- encourage OM to finish sentences, e.g. wash your face. This was used by the nurses and occupational therapist in activities of daily living.

Receptive skills improved rapidly, but spontaneous expression returned slowly, leaving OM with dyspraxic speech that was often unintelligible to the listener. The following goals were then set:

- continued encouragement of use of gestures and facial expression;
- encourage OM to slow down speech;
- feedback when speech not understood, in order to encourage OM to monitor and listen to own speech;
- encourage activities/games such as Connect Four, Noughts and Crosses, reading newspapers and magazines. Simple cognitive games are useful in engaging patients in social interaction, developing concentration and attention skills and are immediately rewarding in outcome;
- writing of own and family names, so able to sign cards;
- telling the time, to promote independence and orientation.

OM was seen daily and new goals were set on a weekly basis by the multidisciplinary team.

Outcome: Mild receptive and moderate expressive dysphasia. Mild reading difficulties and moderate writing difficulties. Returned home and continued rehabilitation in a local day hospital. Referral to local Stroke Association. OM's future communication needs will be met by the voluntary sector. The author thinks that needs have been well met by speech–language therapy service, by a combination of direct therapy and close liaison with the relatives who have utilized OM's total communication skills. Also, relatives were encouraged to contact the speech–language therapist following discharge if the situation altered.

FEEDING AND SWALLOWING PROBLEMS

Older people are more at risk of developing feeding and swallowing problems than younger adults, because of the interrelated problems of physical and mental illness. Age-related physiological changes, chronic disease and medication can influence:

- swallowing function;
- behavioural and cognitive function;
- ability to self feed.

These problems can lead to additional problems:

- dehydration;
- inadequate nutrient intake;
- chest infection/aspiration pneumonia.

Swallowing problems are not uncommon in the older population. The incidence of dysphagia secondary to stroke is reported to range from 25 to 40%, depending on the methodology of data collection (Gordon, Hewer and Wade, 1987; Veis and Logemann, 1985). Progressive neurological disease and organic brain disorder, which are most prevalent in the older population, are also well recognized for contributing to dysphagia and feeding disorders. Feinberg et al. (1990) conclude that dysphagia in the elderly is due to neuromuscular disease, debilitation, dementia, depression and structural abnormality.

Many older people are prescribed a variety of medications which may have an adverse effect on eating practice and swallowing function (Weiden and Harrigan, 1986). Some drugs affect nutritional intake by impairing the appetite, causing nausea and altering the sense of taste. Sedative drugs, or those that cause disorientation and confusion, can have a significant influence on swallowing. Medication which has an action or side effect of diminishing oral secretions can result in drying of the oral and pharyngeal mucosae and adversely influence swallowing in three main ways:

- reduction of saliva to bind food particles to form a bolus;
- reduction of saliva to lubricate the oral cavity (this aids oral transit and protects the oral mucosa);
- inhibition of the swallowing 'reflex'.

Anti-psychotic drugs are known to contribute to dystonia and tardive dyskinesis. Movement disorders of the face, jaw and tongue interfere with the initiation and control of mastication and swallowing.

Oropharyngeal dysphagia (or difficulty with chewing and swallowing) affects both the voluntary and the automatic aspects of the oral–pharyngeal swallowing function and this may deteriorate or be lost when not practised for even relatively brief periods.

PROBLEMS ASSOCIATED WITH DYSPHAGIA

Aspiration is known to occur during sleep in the normal population (Huxley *et al.*, 1978). However, if lung function is impaired, then the risk of pneumonia increases with either single or recurrent episodes of aspiration. Aspiration is known to account for 6% of deaths following stroke in ambulant survivors (Elliott, 1988).

Dysphagia and severe malnutrition causing admission to hospital carries a 13% risk of mortality, regardless of aetiology (Sitzman, 1990). It is known that nutritional state influences both length of stay and eventual outcome in the older patient (Cederholm and Hellstrom, 1992; Unosson *et al.*, 1994). Not only does dysphagia contribute to mortality and morbidity, but also to psychosocial complications such as social isolation and embarrassment (Emick-Herring and Wood, 1990).

MANAGEMENT OF FEEDING AND SWALLOWING DISORDERS

Dysphagia is now recognized as an important consequence of neurological illness (Whitaker and Romer, 1993). Early identification of swallowing problems is essential in reducing mortality and morbidity and in minimizing psychological sequelae such as fear, embarrassment and social isolation. In some conditions swallowing problems are not evident at the time of the diagnosis of the disease, but as the disease progresses swallowing function can become severely impaired. Some patients exhibit dysphagia as the first and only sign of their disease, while others experience dysphagia in a constellation of other signs and symptoms, which makes it difficult to determine to what extent dysphagia is contributing to morbidity and mortality.

A systematic approach to assessment is essential and should be tailored to individual needs. However, the patient's needs are often complex and management requires a co-ordinated multidisciplinary approach with both patient and relatives. In our acute and community hospitals the core team members most often called upon for advice are:

- Speech–language therapists, whose main responsibility is often to co-ordinate the dysphagia rehabilitation programme;
- Dietitians, who make recommendations regarding nutritional needs, the use of supplements and non-oral feeding methods and regimes. The dietitian is also a useful resource in ensuring that the patient's nutritional needs are in line with ethnic dietary habits and practice (see also Chapter 15);
- Nursing staff, who are often the ones who, on the ward, initially identify swallowing or feeding problems. They are also responsible for monitoring the patient's daily nutritional intake, maintaining oral hygiene and supervising eating at mealtimes (see Chapter 10);

- Physiotherapists, who contribute to assessment of swallowi
  patients have a tracheotomy or are ventilated, and assist with po.
  and provide chest physiotherapy (see also Chapter 13);
- Occupational therapists, who assist with adaptive equipment a   ..cip
  to promote independent feeding skills in patients who have visual and
  perceptual impairment (see also Chapter 14);
- The patient's physician, who co-ordinates specialist investigations
  from neurologists and the ear, nose and throat department, etc., and
  contributes to decisions regarding oral/non-oral feeding (see also
  Chapter 2).

The keystone of effective multidisciplinary co-ordination is good communication and liaison.

Case study

HB aged 79 years was admitted to an acute elderly care unit. A
stroke was diagnosed which had resulted in a right hemiplegia,
right-sided neglect, dysphasia and dysphagia. The patient was
referred to speech–language therapy 24 h after admission for assessment and advice regarding both communication and swallowing
difficulties. However, the nursing team felt that the most urgent priority
was to get some idea how they could manage the swallowing problems. Speech–language therapy assessment and observation identified
the following:

- The patient was drowsy but attempted to attend to social contact.
- The chest was clear (according to physiotherapy evaluation).
- At this stage auditory comprehension appeared to be severely
  impaired, but situational understanding was apparent.
- Expressive language was also severely impaired and no speech
  had been heard.
- Assessment of cranial nerves for swallowing indicated the fol-
  lowing level of dysfunction:

  - 7th CN facial nerve, face asymmetrical, affected on right side;
  - 9th CN glossopharyngeal – gag diminished;
  - 10th CN vagus, difficult to determine as no speech available,
    and unable/couldn't cough to command;
  - 12th CN hypoglossal, tongue asymmetrical on protrusion.

Functional swallow – coughed on thin fluids, managed thickened
fluids and puréed food on assessment. However, despite the ability
to swallow some food consistencies safely, she was unable to meet
her nutritional needs without supplements.

Supplements were provided by the dietitian, because of severe fatigue during mealtimes, i.e. she tended to manage only a few teaspoonsful. Case discussion between medical, nursing and therapy staff resulted in the following goals being set.

- An adequate oral diet using appropriate food textures and consistency. This consisted of high-protein puréed diet, thickened fluids and supplements. All oral intake was monitored on a regular basis to ensure nutritional needs were being met.
- Supervised feeding in the early stages of recovery. She was spoon fed by nursing staff.
- Supervised while self feeding. Equipment was provided by occupational therapist to enhance self-feeding skills and independence.
- Weighed weekly.
- Outcome – all swallowing problems resolved over the next 5/6 weeks. Independent with feeding, maintained weight. Remained moderately/severely dysphasic.
- Discharged to slow-stream rehabilitation unit.

REHABILITATION OF THE OLDER PATIENT

The aim of this chapter has been to describe the various impairments the older person may experience as part of the normal ageing process and those due to disease or illness, and to promote the concept of the 'client' or 'customer' centred approach to rehabilitation. Our definition of rehabilitation is to minimize the impact of communication or swallowing disorders on daily living. Active collaboration with other healthcare professionals aids our understanding and drives the need to achieve desired outcomes. Most clinicians will recognize that the focus of 'rehabilitation' will often fall on the relatives and carers, because it is they who will need to understand how best to determine what opportunities the patient has to communicate, and what system they can use to indicate their intention to communicate.

THE FUTURE

Speech–language therapists recognize the need to deliver high-quality services which meet the needs of individual patients, their relatives/carers and other healthcare professionals. Purchasers need professional advice on how to prioritize services and what form of management they should take. An innovative approach to management is needed if we are to continue supplying speech–language therapy services to a growing older population. The use of assistants and the voluntary sector is often considered to be a cheaper resource. Effective training of volunteers and assistants needs to be researched with carefully targeted patient populations, to ensure that an appropriate and effective service is being delivered. Patients with more chronic communication disorders must have access to those who understand their needs, to avoid social isolation and retain mental health. Access to group or individual treatment is essential during the patient's lifetime as situations and lifestyles change. We need to consider carefully how to provide this resource from limited means.

An attractive option is for a speech–language therapist to act as consultant, to assess patients, liaise with primary and secondary healthcare teams, and help design a package of care that fully utilizes assistants, the voluntary sector and social services, to measure outcomes and initiate clinical audits.

REFERENCES

Ball, K.K., Beard, B.L., Roenker, D.L., Miller, R.L. and Griggs, D.S. (1988) Age and visual search: expanding the useful field of view. *Journal of the Optical Society of America*, **5**, 2210–19.

Bayles, K.A., Tomoeda, C.K and Caffrey, J.T. (1982) Language and dementia producing diseases. *Communicative Disorders*, **7**, 131–46.

Bever, T.G. (1970) The cognitive basis for linguistic structures, in *Cognition and the Development of Language* (ed J.R. Hayes), John Wiley & Sons, New York.

Cattel, R.B. (1963) The theory of fluid and crystallized intelligence. *Journal of Educational Psychology*, **54**, 1–22.

Cederholm, T. and Hellstrom, K. (1992) Nutritional status in recently hospitalized and free-living elderly subjects. *Gerontology*, **38**, 105–10.

Clarke, E.O. (1980) Semantic and episodic memory impairment in normal and cognitively impaired elderly adults. *Language and Communication in the Elderly*, Lexington, Massachusetts, DC Heath.

College of Speech and Language Therapists (1991) *Communicating Quality. Professional Standards for Speech and Language Therapists*, Vision Design Group, London.

Darley, F., Aronson, A. and Brown, J. (1975) *Motor Speech Disorders*, Lea & Febiger, Philadelphia.

Davis, G.A. and Wilcox, M.J. (1985) *Adult Asphasia Rehabilitation; Applied Pragmatics*, Nelson, Windsor NFER.

Elliott, J.L. (1988) Swallowing disorders in the elderly: a guide to diagnosis and treatment. *Geriatrics*, **43**, 95–113.

Emick-Herring, B. and Wood, P. (1990) A team approach to neurologically based swallowing disorders. *Rehabilitation Nursing*, **15**, xxx.

Feinberg, R.S., Knebl, J., Tully, J. *et al.* (1990) Aspiration in the elderly. *Dysphagia*, **5**, 61–72.

Gordon, C., Hewer, R. and Wade, D.T. (1987) Dysphagia in acute stroke. *British Medical Journal*, **295**, 411–14.

Gravell, R. (1988) *Communication Problems in Elderly People: Practical Approaches to Managemen*, Croom Helm, London.

Hollien, H. (1987) Old voices: what do we really know about them? *Journal Voice*, **1**(1), 2–17.

Huber, S.J., Shuttleworth, E.C. and Freidenberg, D.L. (1989) Neuropsychological differences between the dementias of Alzheimers and Parkinson's disease. *Archives of Neurology*, **46**, 1287–91.

Huxley, E.J., Viroslav, J., Gray, W.R. *et al.* (1978) Pharyngeal aspiration in normal adults and patients with depressed consciousness. *American Journal of Medicine*, **64**, 564–8.

Jarvik, K. (1962) Biological differences in intellectual functioning. *Vita Humana*, **5**, 195–203.

Knight, R.G. (1992) *The Neuropsychology of Degenerative Brain Diseases*, Lawrence Earlbaum, Hillsdale, New Jersey.

Lieberman, P., Friedman, J. and Feldman, L.S. (1990) Syntax comprehension in Parkinson's disease. *Journal of Nervous and Mental Disease*, **178**, 360–6.

Lubinski, R. (1981) Language and aging: an environmental approach to intervention. *Aspens Systems Corp./Topics in Language Disorders*, **September**, 89–97.

Lubinski, R. (1984) Environmental considerations for institutionalised demented patients. Paper at NYSSHA convention.

Luchsinger, R. and Arnold, G.E. (1965) *Voice, Speech and Language*, Constable, London.

Maccoby, E.E. (1971) Age change in the selective perception of verbal materials, in *The Perception of Language*, Charles E. Merrill, Columbus, Ohio.

Matison, R., Mayeux, R., Rosen, J. and Fahn, S. (1982) 'Tip-of-the-tongue' phenomena in Parkinson's disease. *Neurology*, **32**, 567–70.

Maxim, J. (1982) Language changes with increasing age. *Communication in Elderly People*, Monograph no. 3, College of Speech–Language Therapists, London.

Maxim, J. and Bryan, K. (1994) *Language of the Elderly: A Clinical Perspective*. Whurr Publishers, London.

Murdoch, B.E. (1990) *Acquired Speech and Language Disorders*, Chapman & Hall, London.

Oxtoby, M. (1982) *Parkinson's Disease Patients and their Social Needs*, Parkinson's Disease Society, London.

Rabbitt, P. (1965) An age decrement in the ability to ignore irrelevant information. *Journal of Gerontology*, **20**, 233–8.

Rabbitt, P. (1979) Some experiments and a model for change in attentional selectivity with old age, in *Brain Function in Old Age*, Springer-Verlag, New York.

Robertson, S.J. and Thomson, F. (1983) Speech therapy in Parkinson's disease: a study of the efficacy and long term effects of intensive speech therapy. *British Journal of Disorders of Communication*, **370**, 10–12.

Ross, E.D. (1993) Acute agitation and other behaviours associated with Wernicke aphasia and their possible neurological bases. *Neuropsychiatry, Neuropsychology and Behavioural Neurology*, **6**, 9–18.

Royal College of Physicians Committee on Geriatrics (1981) Organic mental impairment in the elderly. *Journal of the Royal College of Physicians*, **15**, 142–67.

Schonfield, D., Truman, V. and Kline, D. (1982) Recognition tests of dichotic listening and the age variable. *Journal of Gerontology*, **27**, 487–93.

Scott, S. and Caird, F.I. (1983) Speech therapy for Parkinson's disease. *Journal of Neurology, Neurosurgery and Psychiatry*, **46**, 104–44.

Sitzman, J.V. Jr (1990) Nutritional support of the dysphagic patient: methods, risks and complications of therapy. *Journal of Parenteral and Enteral Nutrition*, **14**, 60–3.

Unosson, M., Ek, A.C., Bjurulf, P. *et al.* (1994) Feeding dependence and nutritional status after acute stroke. *Stroke*, **25**(2), 366–71.

Veis, S.L. and Logemann, J.A. (1985) Swallowing disorders in persons with cerebrovascular accident. *Archives of Physical Medicine and Rehabilitation*, **66**, 372–5.

Wahrborg, P. (1991) *Assessment and Management of Emotional and Psychosocial Reactions to Brain Damage and Aphasia*, Far Communications, Leicester.

Wechsler, D. (1985) *The Measurement of Appraisal of Adult Intelligence*, Baillière, Tindall and Cox, New York.

Weiden, P. and Harrigan, M. (1986) A clinical guide for diagnosing and managing patients with drug induced dysphagia. *Hospital Community Psychiatry*, **37**, 3396–8.

Weintraub, S., Rubin, N.P. and Marsel-Mesulam, M.M. (1990) Primary progressive aphasia: longitudinal course, neuropsychological profile and language features. *Archives of Neurology*, **47**, 1329–35.

Whitaker, J. and Romer, J. (1983) The assessment and management of neurogenic swallowing disorders, in *Neurological Rehabilitation* (eds R. Greenward, M.P. Barnes, T.M. MacMillan and C.D. Ward), Churchill Livingstone, Edinburgh.

The role of the nurse in rehabilitation of older people

10

Anne Gale and Jane Gaylard

INTRODUCTION

The fundamental role of nursing today is concerned with restoring health. Assisting patients to overcome their handicaps, by helping them to return function to a part of the body or by optimizing the use of remaining abilities, is the essence of rehabilitation. Historically the term rehabilitation has often been used by nurses in a relatively limited way to describe a specialized area dealing with severely handicapped patients. The underlying philosophy of contemporary nursing, however, is that care is based on planning and using skills that prevent deterioration or restore physical function immediately the patient is admitted to the ward or referred to the community team. Some have termed this rehabilitative nursing care.

WHAT IS NURSING?

Nursing practice involves the application of knowledge and the performance of a variety of skills to improve the level of an individual's health. Nurses use specialist skills with both 'sick' and 'well' individuals. Regardless of the context in which a nurse may work, for example, preventive nursing care (health promotion), care of the terminally ill, or restorative nursing care (rehabilitation), all nurses learn core skills that are fundamental to the practice of nursing. Many definitions of nursing have been proposed by nursing commentators, a reflection of the evolution of nursing practice as health need changes in today's society. The following definition is valued by the authors for its clarity.

> The unique function of the nurse is to assist the individual, sick or well, in the performance of those activities contributing to health or its recovery (or to a peaceful death) that he would perform

unaided if he had the necessary strength, skill or knowledge and to do this in such a way as to help him gain independence as soon as possible.

Henderson, 1966

Henderson's universally accepted definition of nursing clearly identifies the key aim and role of nursing to be that of assisting the individual to be as independent as possible. Henderson identified 14 key areas that applied to the health needs of individuals who require nursing. These are to:

1. breathe normally;
2. eat and drink adequately;
3. eliminate body wastes;
4. move and maintain desirable postures;
5. sleep and rest;
6. select suitable clothing (dress and undress);
7. maintain body temperature within normal range by adjusting clothing and modifying the environment;
8. keep the body clean and groomed and protect the integument;
9. avoid environmental dangers and avoid injury to others;
10. communicate with others in expressing emotions, fear or opinions;
11. worship according to one's faith;
12. work in such a way that there is a sense of accomplishment;
13. play or participate in various forms of recreation;
14. learn, discover, or satisfy the curiosity that leads to normal development and health and the use of available health facilities.

These areas have become identified as the essence of 'basic nursing care' and are considered essential to human welfare.

The concept of basic nursing 'care' is one that often causes debate. Key to this debate is the interpretation that to 'care' for the patient equates with 'doing for' the patient and thus is incompatible with rehabilitation. Whilst 'doing for' patients is undoubtedly an element of the nurses' role, it is by no means limited to this. Orem (1980) has described nurses' helping methods as ranging from providing total help by acting and doing for the individual, to guiding, supporting and providing a therapeutic environment, to teaching other carers. The emphasis laid on caring for patients by 'doing for' them at the expense of the others may well be the tendency of society at large to lay emphasis on 'cure' rather than 'care', curable 'acute' conditions prevailing over 'chronic' conditions. Frequently it is the medically orientated model of nursing care that captures public imagination. As the needs of the population change, so will their demands, but education is needed so that the facilitation of independence through rehabilitation programmes does not result in an assumption of dependence for people with chronic disability. Nurses themselves and their colleagues are largely responsible for the development of this lay view.

Throughout this chapter it is important to remember that care is not to be equated with 'doing for' an individual; rather, the role of the nurse is guiding, supporting, teaching and providing the therapeutic environment to enable rehabilitation to be actively practised. This role will both support and most certainly be sustained by the contribution of other members of the multidisciplinary team.

DEVELOPMENT OF ELDERLY CARE NURSING AS A SPECIALITY

As already described (Chapter 1), the development of geriatric medical care was born out of the attempt to replace the policy of custodial care. Essentially those patients who failed to respond to medical expectation of cure and discharge were re-accommodated in an environment governed by routine and regulation in which the nurses' duty was to provide 24-hour bedside care (Norton, 1977).

A key text in the development of elderly care nursing is *The Nursing of the Elderly Sick* (Rudd, 1954). This provides a concise definition of elderly care nursing that includes the maintenance of physical, mental and social independence, prevention of chronic ill health and the maintenance of the individual in the community rather than an institution as the preferred option. Rudd observed that the change in attitude toward elderly patients from that of custodial care to that of investigative medical treatment and physical mobilization demanded that the needs of the patient as an individual be considered and restoration of function, rather than concentrating on temporary nursing requirements, should be the prime objective of the nurse. This theme was continued in Doreen Norton's research, culminating in the landmark work *An Investigation of Geriatric Nursing Problems in Hospital* (Norton, McLaren and Exton-Smith, 1962) in which three basic areas were identified in which nurses could improve their care of elderly patients:

- individual needs-based patient assessment;
- the grouping of elderly patients on wards according to their identified nursing problems;
- the maintenance of individual nursing records for each patient, to aid communication and evaluation of nursing interventions.

In addition, the authors' model of elderly care nursing featured the systematic study of basic nursing care, the recognition of the importance of the environment as a potential tool of nursing (e.g. design, equipment, etc.) and the requirement to consider the total needs of each patient and to set individual goals.

Norton's 1965 work (cited by Kitson, 1991) considered the relationship between the geriatric medical and nursing models; she proposed that there were two distinct groups of patients in elderly care nursing: those patients with the potential to regain some self-care ability (assessment and rehabilitation patients in medical terms) and those needing nursing care for the rest of their life – the long-stay category. The role of the nurse is to re-enable the first group to self care, so that rather than 'doing for' the patient the nurse aids the patient by teaching appropriate skills and providing emotional support and encouragement. The nurse has a key role in the multidisciplinary team in co-ordinating the team approach, noting conflicting aims and facilitating the resolution to an unambiguous goal. The role of the nurse with those who require continuing care is to 'maintain the delicate balance between giving of tender loving care and the maintenance of the last vestiges of independence' (Kitson, 1991).

EDUCATION

The recognition of rehabilitation of the older person as a nursing speciality has been enhanced by the provision of further education and training for nurses. This is seen as necessary to inform nurses of the skills and knowledge that they require to be effective in a rehabilitation setting. All nurses caring for older people needing rehabilitation should have participated in a course such as the Care and Rehabilitation of the Physically Disabled Adult. This course in outline is one approved by the nurses' controlling body for education (in England, the English National Board, with similar national boards for Scotland, Wales and Northern Ireland). Similarly, schools of nursing offer many other courses for qualified and unqualified staff exploring many aspects of nursing that enhance rehabilitation of the older person. The acknowledgement by the nursing profession that rehabilitation nursing requires further education has been a key factor that has enabled many elderly care units to develop innovative programmes of care that now make this branch of nursing a leader in nursing developments.

ELDERLY CARE NURSING TODAY

The following example of an Elderly Care Unit nursing philosophy illustrates how the fundamental beliefs expressed by Norton are integral to today's nursing.

The nursing care offered within Elderly Services is based on the belief that it is the right of each patient to be cared for in a manner that recognises and values his/her individuality.

A systematic approach to patient assessment and establishment of realistic goals of care is therefore employed with, or on behalf of, each individual patient. The aim of nursing care is to promote the optimum state of health and independence.

Patients and their carers are encouraged to participate in goal-setting and share decision-making. Regular and accurate information shared between nursing staff, patients and carers is acknowledged to be crucial to this process.

A 'named nurse' (i.e. Primary Nurse) is allocated to each patient from admission to discharge. The Primary Nurse is responsible for managing all aspects of nursing care including information sharing. Nursing care is planned in conjunction with medical and therapy staff.

A commitment to the employment of high calibre nursing staff, continuous in-service training based on up-to-date research findings relating to elderly care nursing, in addition to regular supervision of staff, ensures the delivery of high quality nursing care commensurate with national and local professional standards.

At all time the patient's rights to privacy, dignity and confidentiality are upheld.

(*Philosophy of Nursing: Elderly Services*, Southampton Community Hospitals Trust, 1995; unpublished)

THE ORGANIZATION OF REHABILITATION SERVICES FOR THE OLDER PATIENT

Essentially there are three basic ways in which treatment and care is organizationally delivered to the older person: as a hospital in-patient, as a day patient, or in the person's own residence. Nurses may practise in any of these environments. Any one of these has its advantages and disadvantages, but choice is dependent on the needs of the patient, together with facilities available in the health care district.

It has been argued that the organization of professional hospital-centred care for the older person receives disproportionate attention compared with care delivery in other settings (Evers, 1986). It is important, however, to recognize the contribution that traditional hospital-based geriatric departments have made in raising the status of older people and their potential for rehabilitation, and the role such departments have in the education of healthcare professionals. Whether they can sustain their influence in general medical and/or community-based care is the future challenge.

IN-PATIENT CARE

Rehabilitation services for older in-patients are still largely situated in departments of geriatric medicine, a reflection of the historical origins of geriatric medicine being rooted in the acute medical model of care. Where beds are physically situated inevitably has implications on the staffing, resources and therapeutic environment that may be created. Where beds are provided in a single unit, two main patterns of organization are frequently described: multi-purpose wards and single-purpose wards. Multi-purpose wards cater for patients requiring short-term assessment and therapy facilities, extended care and rehabilitation over a longer period of time. Single-purpose wards are organized to provide facilities dedicated to one type of the aforementioned patient groups. In addition to these two basic patterns of organization, some hospitals utilize units based on specific diagnostic groups, e.g. stroke or orthopaedics. It is argued that single-purpose wards allow for effective use of resources and enable the environment to be appropriately designed for its prime use. Whilst this may be advantageous to assessment and rehabilitation patients, the problems of institutionalization, depersonalization and the relative lack of professional expertise described by many researchers of elderly long-stay care environments may not be ameliorated by this separatist approach.

DAY HOSPITAL CARE

Day hospitals originated from the need to provide clinical team management of patients without the need for the person to be hospitalized. The essential difference between day hospitals and rehabilitative out-patient facilities is that day hospitals provide an integrated multidisciplinary service to the patient, rather than a series of fragmented episodes of rehabilitation with separate elements of the service. There are many issues to be addressed in the use of day hospitals, and clarity over objectives, criteria and staff roles will go some way towards successful working.

HOME FROM HOSPITAL SCHEMES

Such schemes are often developed with the local authority social services department to enable early and successful discharge by providing traditional hospital-based services in the patient's own home when they are at their most vulnerable during the early phase of the discharge. Schemes vary in their scope as a result of local circumstances.

ORGANIZATION OF THE HOSPITAL NURSING TEAM

Regardless of the environment, nursing staff are essentially organized in teams, whether on a ward or in a day hospital. The team comprises a combination of trained nurses and unqualified staff, supervised by qualified nurses. The team is led by a nursing sister or ward manager, who is responsible for the overall management and organization of nursing staff; this includes ensuring that the skill mix employed on the ward is appropriate to the needs of the client.

Historically a number of methods of organizing nursing care have been used by nurses.

'Task' nursing, where specific nursing tasks, for example, doing all the observations, are allocated to a nurse;

'Team' nursing, where all of a patient's care is allocated to one nurse for the duration of a shift;

'Primary nursing', where a patient is allocated to a trained nurse for their duration of stay in that care environment.

Whilst all three modes of organizing nursing care can be observed to some degree in contemporary nursing, primary nursing is further described here as it has been (arguably) largely developed and has enjoyed most success in elderly care nursing settings. In addition, primary nursing is advocated by many as the method for organizing care, as it best facilitates the desired individualized and holistic approach to patient care.

PRIMARY NURSING

Although there are variations described by authors in the practice and implementation of primary nursing, the principles remain the same, as described by its originator Manthey (1980, p. 31).

1. Allocation and acceptance of responsibility for decision making to one individual;
2. Individual assignment of daily care by case method;

3. Direct person-to-person communication;
4. One person operationally responsible for the quality of care administered to patients on a unit 24 hours a day, 7 days a week.

Primary nursing is then a systematic way of organizing the nursing team on the ward. Patients are divided into groups; each group is allocated to a specific nurse called a 'primary nurse'. The primary nurse has responsibility for assessing, planning and evaluating care for the group of patients from their admission to their discharge. Each primary nurse also acts as an 'associate nurse' for groups of patients other than her own. As an associate nurse, she has the responsibility only for implementing care planned by the primary nurse when she is not on duty (Manthey, 1988).

ORGANIZATION OF NURSING CARE IN THE COMMUNITY

District nurses may be organized geographically or 'attached' to one or more GP practices and they are responsible for the nursing care of the patients therein. The district nurse is currently usually employed by the NHS Trust to provide nursing care to people in their own home, health centre or residential accommodation, but other models are being developed.

The work of the District Nursing Service is, in essence, the assessment and delivery of care and support to patients and carers in their homes. Patients will normally have been referred by the GP and may just have been discharged from hospital. Patients may be 'on the books' for, at one extreme, only one visit, or, at the other, for many years (Kelly and O'Leary, 1992, p. 9). The management of the workload of the district nursing teams is a crucial part of the role of the district nurse:

> The district nurse is the leader of the district nursing team within the primary health care services. Working with her may be registered general nurses (RGN's), enrolled nurses (EN's) and the nursing auxiliaries (NA). The district nurse delegates as appropriate to EN's who can thus have their own case load, but who remain wholly accountable to the district nurse for the care that they give to patient ...
>
> *Mackenzie, 1989, p. 10*

Mackenzie (1989, p. 20) goes on to describe the required skills of the district nurse thus:

> Many of the skills used in management are practised every day by the district nurse and are an integral part of her role. By definition she is the leader of the nursing team. Effective leadership means that the district nurse has to initiate new ideas, motivate staff, establish

effective communication systems, identify staff potential and enable all members of the team to function at their full potential. At the very least the district nurse has to manage a caseload, as detailed in the CNO letter (DHSS, 1977), and has responsibilities for patient care in relation to other staff. Within this responsibility she has to make referrals, delegate (with the appropriate accountability and responsibility), make decisions often in emergency situations without immediate recourse to medical advice, identify gaps in provision of services, utilise resources and evaluate the effectiveness of nursing care.

Kelly and O'Leary's (1992) study acknowledged that the following caseload management issues are often not addressed in district nursing.

- Type and number of cases referred;
- Length of time patients are on the books and why;
- Effectiveness of care and treatment regimes;
- Effectiveness of planning and routing of visits;
- Matching of the grade of the nurse to the needs of the patient.

The main reasons given for this is the absence or inadequacies of information systems and the heavy visiting loads of senior grades of staff (G and H grades). Senior grade nurses felt they were unable to devote appropriate amounts of time to management of care issues, e.g. careful monitoring of individual plans of care, or discussion of the delivery and progress of care on a systematic basis with junior members of staff. The main reasons for this were heavy (but often inappropriate) caseloads (Kelly and O'Leary, 1992). The increasing need in the future will be the need for district nurses to more closely plan and evaluate the effectiveness, appropriateness and duration of the nursing service that provides certain types of care. District nurses will have to consider the contribution to the care plan that the patient or carers can take on and where other agencies may provide a more appropriate service. The issue of a more generic style of working also has to be addressed, especially where multi-skilling of staff of different disciplines enables a more cost-effective approach, so long as back-up expert help is available.

Political influence over the last decade in relation to health care delivery has had a significant effect on nursing care. Hospital-based nurses now have less time to make decisions regarding care options and district nurses, as a result (particularly since the 1993 enactment of the Community Care Act), have a greater number of complex care decisions to make, since their clients are discharged earlier in their recovery phase and increasing numbers of elderly are nursed in the community. The employment and management of appropriately skilled nursing staff is the current challenge to district nursing, as traditional community nursing tasks are increasingly done by unqualified staff from other statutory or privately owned concerns, as a result of competitive tendering. Communication between such plural providers is even more important, to ensure consistency and avoid gaps and duplication.

NURSING ASSESSMENT OF PATIENT NEED

Regardless of the environment where the patient is nursed, the 'nursing process' is the framework used by nurses to assess, plan, implement and evaluate patients' nursing care. A number of definitions exist, for example 'the application of scientific problem-solving to nursing care' (Marriner, 1983), or 'a systematic method of decision making and planning nursing care' (McFarlane and Castledine, 1982). Whatever definition is preferred, all tend to suggest a planned, methodical and organized process of critical reflective thought (Prophit, 1980).

NURSING ASSESSMENT

The assessment element of the nursing process has been usefully described as having two phases: firstly, collecting information about the patient and his situation and secondly, assessing the patient's needs, difficulties and problems noted from the aforementioned information. Problems are then prioritized according to hierarchy of importance, wherever possible with the patient (French, 1983). The aim of nursing assessment, therefore, is:

- to assess the patient risk (and maintain life in emergency situations);
- to establish rapport;
- to collect information used to plan nursing care;
- to review and interpret the patient's health state;
- to determine what problems exist;
- to establish a baseline for the patient's health state (for monitoring of improvement/deterioration);
- to identify the patient's level of understanding.

Collecting the information required for nursing assessment is achieved by a number of routes; interviewing or observation may be used. With encouragement, problems may be expressed by the patient, their family or another health care professional in addition to nursing staff. Patient dependence scores may be used to describe the patient's 'baseline' state and then to delegate appropriate nursing staff to manage the patient's needs. In many units this information is collected on a centralized database, to which all health care professionals can contribute and have access, and should enable varying dependency to be met with responsive staffing allocation unit wide.

PLANNED NURSING CARE

The nursing plan consists of a number of nursing strategies designed to resolve or minimize the problems identified during assessment. Each plan is documented as a 'nursing care plan' and is a specific and concise record of individualized care designed for each specific problem identified as experienced by that specific patient. Goals of care (i.e. anticipated outcomes) are identified with the patient and recorded on the care plan before care is implemented. An evaluation time/date is estimated, agreed and recorded, appropriate to the proposed strategy of care.

It is recognized that the nursing plan is only a part of the patient's over-all rehabilitation plan, and this is taken into account. The rehabilitation team may agree a goal of sitting balance, for example, so that the patient can perform the basic activities he might wish to do in that position. Whilst the physiotherapist might outline the plan, the nursing staff would be instrumental in carrying this through with the other members of the team. Conversely, problems relating to continence, for example, may be planned for in detail by nursing staff who, whilst dealing with the problem the majority of the time, would need the input of other health care workers. Increasingly nurses, together with the patient, carer and the rest of the multidisciplinary rehabilitation team, are contributing to collaborative care plans, i.e. joint care plans. This can produce a more co-ordinated and purposeful treatment plan from the perspective of the patient, who may be able more clearly to understand how each element of their rehabilitation programme effects their overall goals of treatment and care.

IMPLEMENTATION OF NURSING CARE

Delivery of nursing care, i.e. the implementation phase of the nursing process, is undertaken by trained professional nurses with the support of supervised unqualified staff. Contributions from learner nurses or untrained staff are carefully monitored by qualified nurses.

EVALUATION OF NURSING CARE

Evaluation of care, the fourth element of the nursing process, is made against the agreed goals of care by the qualified nurse within the time-frame agreed.

It can be seen that the nursing process is a dynamic activity, which requires continuous evaluation and re-evaluation, dependent on the changing status of the patient. The contribution of the patient in all aspects of the nursing process is also dynamic, and clearly the capacity of some patients to be able to participate in care is greater than that of others.

MODELS OF NURSING

To provide comprehensive care, the nurse uses skills that involve application of the sciences such as anatomy, physiology, pathology, sociology and psychology. These, together with nursing theory and research, form the foundation of nursing knowledge.

A number of nursing 'models' (i.e. nursing theories) exist that provide nurses with a basis on which to organize their assessment and subsequent planning of care with the patient. Whilst it is beyond the scope of this chapter to discuss individual nursing models in detail, generally they share common themes or concepts that propose a systematic basis for application of the nursing process. These include the nature of the individual, society, or the environment for care, the nature of health and the role of nursing. The findings of the assessment are interpreted according to the model used. Nursing models have been devised inductively and/or deductively, that is to say the theories outside of nursing have been applied to nursing (induction), and introduced to the individual nursing model together with the theorist's own experience and observations in nursing (deduction).

There are three models of nursing that appear eminently suitable for the rehabilitation setting.

- Roper, Logan and Tierney (1985) recommended the use of the activities of living as a major emphasis, together with the progression along the lifespan and the dependence/independence continuum. The three main nursing activities are preventive, comforting or seeking, the last being a search for answers to problems presented by patients and the care that they require.
- Orem's (1980) model of care focuses on the concept of self care. This is related to the belief that people have a desire to take responsibility for their own health care and that this is a basic human need. This model also incorporates developmental self-care requisites which involves changes during the life-cycle of the individual. Health deviation self-care requisites arise as a result of illness or disability and demand changes in self-care behaviour. The nursing systems needed to care for individuals are wholly compensatory, partially compensatory or educative and/or supportive in nature.
- Roy's (1976) model is based in psychological theory and focuses on the ability of an individual to adapt to changes in stimuli, be these from within the person or from external circumstances. The model takes into account focal stimuli that may arise from the immediate circumstance such as ill health or bereavement. The other immediate surroundings or contextual stimuli, such as temperature or ward ambience, also affect the ability of an individual to adapt to these

circumstances. Finally, the residual stimuli or beliefs, attitudes and traits that determine individual behaviour are the third element to affect a person's ability to cope with changed circumstances. Assessment must explore the physiological factors, the self-concept that the person has, their function within the family and the wider social sphere and lastly the interdependence between the person and others.

Elements of all these three models are found within nursing rehabilitation settings and may form a useful foundation for nursing care. Aspects of the activities of daily living may form the focus of multidisciplinary interventions. Self-care or adaptation to disability are two other key features of the nurse's role in assisting people to adjust to changes in their lifestyle or circumstance.

All nursing models define in one way or another the environment, the patient or client, the nurse and nursing and lastly health. The importance of these are that the way in which the nurse especially views them will determine the nursing approach to the patients' experience.

THE ENVIRONMENT

The environment and the patient are inseparable in rehabilitation. The ability to achieve any degree of self care is partly determined by this relationship. The nurse in institutional settings therefore has the responsibility to create a therapeutic environment that is conducive to rehabilitation, with the goal of achieving self care or adaptation, where possible. Care provided in the patient's own home, whilst not under the control of the nurse, may require that the nurse encourage an atmosphere promoting self care, so that the patient regains independence.

Clearly the provision of equipment within the hospital setting should be suitable to the promotion of independence. The requirement to be an advocate for other people demands that not only the equipment but also the care provision is centred around the person. The provision of choices with regards to their daily care needs, diet, times of getting up and going to bed are also fundamental to an environment that promotes rehabilitation. The nurse as the person responsible for care provision on a 24-hour basis must also liaise with other professionals for the provision of specialist equipment that will enhance the quality of life for the individual as and when necessary. At home the provision of equipment and structural changes will take much longer to provide, so that adaptation and maintenance of a positive attitude towards rehabilitation will not infrequently be the responsibility of the nurse. Regardless of the physical environment for care delivery, it is essential that the patient's carers (if there are any) and their needs are incorporated into any plan of care.

THE PERSON

Belief that the individual has the potential ability to meet their own self-care needs or alternatively to adapt to differing circumstances, given the right support and intervention must also be a prerequisite in rehabilitation nursing. The ability to allow people to take control of their own lives and provide them with choices must be integral to the nursing plan. Their involvement in decision making can only enhance people's chances to regain independence, the primary goal of rehabilitation (see also Chapter 4).

NURSING

Nursing models identify the functions of the nurse; in the rehabilitation setting these must be moving away from wholly or partially compensatory nursing to an educative or supportive role. The nurse must enable the person to adapt their living activities to their changed circumstances. This may involve seeking innovative ways of achieving these goals.

HEALTH

It is not intended to define health here or to explore the difficulties of this. However, it is important that the nursing care given includes an aspiration for the individual to achieve maximum wellness, given their personal circumstances. Respect for the individual is probably the best starting point for this to be achieved (see also Chapter 4).

THE NURSING ROLE IN THE CARE OF THE OLDER PATIENT

It has been suggested that whilst many nurses work in rehabilitation settings their contribution to the rehabilitation process is still unclear (Waters, 1986). Given the 24-hour presence of nursing it is evident that nurses have a considerable contribution to make to patient rehabilitation. The Royal College of Nursing (1991) suggest that while the role of the nurse in rehabilitation is broad, there is a core part of the process for which nursing responsibility and expertise is held:

- personal hygiene
- skin care
- bowels
- bladder
- wound care
- nutritional intake
- prevention of complications.

The first four items on the list are sometimes regarded as the routine/basic work, but this is to ignore the skills demanded of the nurse and the importance of these areas of care to the clients. An unpublished study by S. Kennedy and N. Zepke in 1983 (RCN, 1991) compared the priorities of therapists and their patients and found that the qualities of helping the patient relax and appreciate their feelings as an individual were considered far more important by patients than the use of technical procedures and decision making: the reverse of the therapist's perceptions.

It is suggested that assisting the patient to have a positive attitude to these 'basic' aspects of clinical care often enables the nurse to have a unique role in rehabilitation, as it is through this intimate care that the nurse–client relationship develops (RCN, 1991). It is important that the nurse takes time to develop rapport with the patient, that the patient's participation in care is encouraged by the nurse and that the patient's perceptions are at the centre of goal setting and care planning. The research findings of Wright (1990) and Jewell (1994) support the belief that the intimate relationship between nurse and patient enables the patient to participate meaningfully in care.

Initially the nursing given to patients by the nurse will provide the care that the persons cannot achieve for themselves. This may meet their immediate needs, but the role of the nurse in rehabilitation is to encourage and enable the patients gradually to take on the responsibility for their own activities of daily living. There can be no prescriptive pathway that determines this transition from providing care to enabling the patient to meet their own needs at an optimal level. Indeed, it would seem to be essential that the role of the nurse in rehabilitation is clearly defined for the patients, to enable them to understand and fully participate in this transition. It also helps to avoid the cultural perceptions that surround the image of the nurse always providing the care (Sheppard, 1994). Where possible the patient's family or carers will share in the rehabilitation programme. Education of the carers by the nurse and the multidisciplinary team is essential, to ensure that optimal practices are consistently maintained.

The 'structured dependence' of old age has been well defined by Townsend (1986), who stated that the dependency of the elderly was the result of societal manufacture – enforced retirement, the imposition of low income, the lack of rights of self determination within institutional settings and, lastly, the fact that community care provision was constructed on the assumption that the recipients were predominantly passive. These societal structures of dependence have created the notion of the 'burden' of caring for older people, rather than the 'challenge'. The role of the rehabilitation nurse is especially important in preserving the rights of the older person and ensuring that they are active decision makers in their own care provision.

CORE SKILLS OF NURSING

PERSONAL HYGIENE

The cleansing, washing, manicure, pedicure and grooming activities of everyday living fall within the responsibility of the nurse. Whilst these are often viewed as menial tasks with little importance, they are in fact procedures by which the nurse may strongly enhance the rehabilitation process for the patient (see also Chapter 11). Maslow (1943) clearly showed that the most basic needs must be met before progression can be undertaken. It is in the encouragement of the person, finding ways of enabling them to meet their own needs, that the process of rehabilitation can be made understandable as well as realizable for the individual. These activities are important for most people to have an acceptable quality of life and so form an ideal basis on which to build a rehabilitation programme. For example, they enable people to choose their clothes and provide guidance to teach them the adaptations they might need to make in order to dress themselves. This is done in association with the occupational therapists (see also Chapter 14), the nurse re-enforcing and reminding people of these skills throughout the 24 hours.

SKIN CARE

The importance of protecting skin from the damage caused by pressure or incontinence is another important aspect of the nurse's role. Assessment of the risk of pressure sore development, first devised in geriatric wards by Norton, McLaren and Exton-Smith (1962), remains if anything more important today, with the increasing frailty associated with the very old and disabled.

Assessment alone is not sufficient; a nurse having identified a person potentially at risk of developing a decubitus ulcer must implement a plan of care that reduces this risk to the minimal achievable. This plan must be founded on sound research evidence and involvement of the continence advisor (see Chapter 15), and should identify the appropriate pressure-relieving devices, as well as suitable regimes to move and position the patient which both promote rehabilitation and minimize the risk of skin damage. Promoting continence and the effective management of incontinence ensure that the skin is not damaged by urine. This is not just another feature of good skin care, but a key feature of promoting the dignity and well being of people. The importance of adequate nutrition and hydration is also essential to skin integrity. In conjunction with the patient and dietitian, the nurse devises an optimal plan of care to promote patient well being (see also Chapter 15). Nursing care must also include other knowledge with regard to pathological conditions and medication that may also be implicated in the development of pressure sores; liaison between the nurse and the pharmacist is invaluable in this respect (see also Chapter 15).

BLADDER AND BOWEL FUNCTION

Another less glamorous but crucial aspect of nursing responsibility is the management of bladder and bowel function. The importance of the maintenance of a comfortable and dignified individual cannot be underestimated. Good assessment throughout the 24 hours enables the nurse to be in the forefront of identifying likely causes of dysfunction, thus enabling appropriate remedial action to be taken, or if this is not possible to provide the highest standards of personal hygiene so that people remain dry and comfortable. The nurse is best placed to monitor oral intake in relation to elimination, either with the patient or on their behalf, if they are unable to do this for themselves. This ability to monitor and assess should guarantee that incontinence is restricted to those for whom there is no cure or remedy. Again, communication with the multi-disciplinary team who will be supervising intake and elimination in different settings throughout the day is essential.

PREVENTION OF COMPLICATIONS

This responsibility demands knowledge of physiological processes and the understanding of diseases and the effects of the multiple pathologies that can affect the very old. The prevention of joint deformity, together with the correct positioning to avoid nerve damage, pain and disordered limb function are essentially a nursing responsibility, as they provide care over a 24-hour period. The prevention of respiratory and circulatory complications, which includes appropriate passive exercise or the promotion of mobility, also requires care over the 24 hours. Rehabilitation demands that complications are prevented and functions are restored.

RISK TAKING IN NURSING

Nursing work has changed considerably over the last two or three decades, and this is likely to continue in the latter part of this century as the nursing role expands to accommodate professional, political and societal influences. As the boundaries of what nursing is seen to be shifts, the individual nurse's world shifts also and, as a consequence, clinical risk taking becomes increasingly part of that world. Running risks can involve exposing the patient or the nurse to the possibility of injury, failure or loss. The future challenge for nurses will be in accurately analysing risk and allocation of resources. Reduced resources could mean that in some instances no intervention is safer than a little intervention, the quality of which may be dubious. This will be a difficult but necessary fact of life for nurses to address. Risk taking may seem a contradiction to this need to prevent complications. Encouraging people to walk independently after the team has minimized the risk does not eliminate the possibility of a fall, but may be a risk worth taking to improve the patient's confidence. The conflict between protecting patients and the need to promote independence, with the resultant risks that may ensue, must be considered and thoroughly documented. Furthermore, the individual concerned and the carer must be involved in those risk taking decisions and should clearly understand both the nature and possible consequences of the action proposed.

In any rehabilitation setting it is imperative that a philosophy with regard to risk taking is developed, in order that the multidisciplinary team is working together to promote independence and all are aware of the risks that could result from these decisions. Relatives, as well, need to be involved and aware that these decisions are designed to improve the quality of life for the person, even though to some this may not seem to be the priority. Risk taking means that the quality of life is a major theme in the care provided, together with the provision for individuals to take control of their lives.

NUTRITIONAL AND FLUID INTAKE

Ensuring that patients are eating and drinking adequately is a nursing responsibility. In institutional settings, the choices available from menus, whilst limited, should be adequate to meet nutritional requirements. The involvement of the dietitian at an early stage of the patient's rehabilitation is important if the nurse, having assessed the patient, notes a nutritional deficit (see Chapter 15). However, the setting in which the food is eaten is also of importance, with the nurse needing to provide an environment conducive to the enjoyment of food and drink. Other family members can also be encouraged to play a role in obtaining favourite foods or drinks, within any dietary constraints, when these are not available within the institution.

MEDICATION

Giving medication to patients is another responsibility that within hospitals may be part of the routine. In the rehabilitation setting the nurse must establish programmes that allow patients to self medicate when able to do so. This ensures that the programme of rehabilitation achieves optimal self care for the individual. The role of the pharmacist is crucial to the success of self-medication programmes: to ensure that labelling and packaging is appropriate to the specific needs of the individual, that drug information is given clearly and that, where used, the same compliance aids are available when the patient is discharged back to the community (see also Chapter 15).

MOTIVATION

The prolonged contact that individuals have with nursing staff in the provision of these aspects of intimate care enables the nurses to establish an affective relationship with the person having rehabilitation. The use of effective listening skills provides an opportunity for nurses to gain insight and understanding and to identify personal differences. This might indicate strategies that may be utilized to improve the motivation for an individual. The complexity of personal circumstances and individual differences must be incorporated into any plan of care if it is to be successful. The guidance and support provided by the multidisciplinary team, notably the medical social worker (Chapter 12), occupational therapist (Chapter 14) and counsellor and clinical psychologist (Chapter 5), will be used by the nurse. Motivation is enhanced by the ongoing support and guidance that nurses are able to give on a regular and ongoing basis. The activities of daily living that need consideration in a rehabilitation programme are the opportunities for this support to be provided.

THE MULTIDISCIPLINARY REHABILITATION TEAM

The hospital-based nurse is an integral and key member of the multidisciplinary team. Within that team the rehabilitation nurse may function as the patient's advocate and mentor (see Chapter 4), and often have responsibility for co-ordination of the differing aspects of the rehabilitation programme offered by the team members. Planning for discharge with the patient and their family or carers will begin early on, as part of the patient's assessment (Jewell, 1993).

The role of the community nurse in this scenario will be to continue the programme of rehabilitation initiated in the hospital. With primary led care, this will change to more activity in the community, with recourse to hospitals an exception. The community nurse is unlikely as yet to have the level of multidisciplinary team support that her hospital colleagues have to hand. Whilst the therapeutic skills of physiotherapy, occupational therapy and speech therapy are available in the community, the skill mix and efficiency measures may make team involvement difficult, with more responsibility falling to community nursing, demanding that district nurses take on additional education and training (see Chapter 1).

The community nurse's patient is more likely to be suffering from chronic disability and the assessments he/she undertakes are commonly

related to long-standing problems and goal setting focused on maintenance of ability and avoidance of secondary problems. While the
hospital nurse has the task of creating a nursing environment that, while
conducive to rehabilitation, also meets the standards laid down in the
Health and Safety at Work Act, the community nurse has to remember
that he/she is a guest in the patient's home and is reliant on the patient
and family's co-operation in achieving safe practice.

In addition, the hospital nurse has support from various services
within the hospital and reasonable access to resources. The community
nurse needs to apply to social service fund holders and GPs in order to
access resources for their patients. Dunnell and Dobbs (1982) identified
that district nurses spend 75% of their time with older clients. One of the
key roles of the district nurse is rehabilitative care or 'tertiary prevention', as Caplan (1961) described it. This is defined as the measures
taken to alleviate an existing condition, prevent complications and
modify the effects of illness. Practical examples of this might include the
following.

- Continuing or implementing a rehabilitation programme for the
  aftercare of stroke patients at home, helping adjustment to
  disability and handicap;
- Teaching safety measures in the home;
- Teaching the client about environmental hazards that contribute
  to poor health (e.g. cold, muscle wasting from immobility,
  preventing constipation, and so on);
- Teaching carers techniques for moving and handling, skin care,
  prevention of pressure sores;
- Aiding drug compliance.

The link between hospital and community is ideally filled by the liaison
nurse, whose role is to interpret the final evaluation of hospital-based team
interventions and relate these to the long-term goals of the patient, in order
to facilitate the community team's assessment and planning of care.
Responsibility for funding these posts is one that neither the hospital nor
the community Trust has been keen to own. This can lead to dissonance
between the government ideal of 'seamless transition of care' and reality.
In areas where agreement has not been met, these posts have become
increasingly under threat and may need intervention by the commissioning authority, who will seek objective evidence of need and measures of
success. On a positive note, some Trusts are endeavouring to bridge this
gap by introducing more specialist nurses.

THE ROLE OF SPECIALIST NURSES

These nurses divide their time between hospital and community and are in an ideal position to act as liaison between hospital and community services in those aspects of care in which they hold specialist knowledge. They are not usually responsible for assessing planning and implementing care, but are primarily a resource for their colleagues who may be endeavouring to implement programmes of rehabilitation for elderly patients in specialities as various as medicine, surgery trauma or oncology.

The rehabilitation nurse may refer laterally for advice from colleagues such as the diabetic, continence, stoma or rheumatology nurse specialist. Rehabilitation goals concentrate on aspects of social skills and functions patients fulfilled before their illness. However, the rehabilitation nurse in elderly care settings needs to be aware that the normal physiological process of ageing will produce effects that no amount of rehabilitation will be able to ameliorate.

THE FUTURE

Older people are major consumers of healthcare. The developments in medical technology, increased life expectancy of the population and social expectations create an increasing demand for healthcare provision. This compounds the problems of the resource-limited statutory services. One of the responsibilities of the present government has been the provision of healthcare services to the (increasingly) older population. Demand is now in real danger of outstripping supply.

The nurse along with other members of the multidisciplinary team, the patient and significant others must develop plans of care that are adjusted to these realities and do not promise that which society is now unable to deliver.

Nevertheless, the nurse, in conjunction with members of the multi-disciplinary team, is a key player in ensuring that community care is achieved. Nurses' extended and frequent contact with the patient often leads to their being the persons most fully aware of all the factors that may affect provision and receipt of care. The nurse must, therefore, whatever the environmental setting for care provision, maintain a strong voice as the older patient's advocate, to ensure that their reasonable demands and expectations are met.

REFERENCES

Caplan, G. (1961) *An Approach to Community Mental Health*, Tavistock, London.
DHSS (1977) *Nursing in Primary Health Care*, Circular CNO (77) 8 DHSS, London.
Dunnell, K. and Dobbs, J. (1982) *Nurses Working in the Community*, Office of

Population Censuses and Surveys, London.

Evers, H.K. (1986) Care of the elderly sick in the UK, in *Nursing Elderly People* (ed S. Redfern), Churchill Livingstone, Edinburgh.

French, P. (1983) *Social Skills of Nursing Practice*, Croom Helm, London.

Henderson, V. (1966) *The Nature of Nursing: A Definition and its Implications for Practice, Research and Education*, Macmillan, New York.

Jewell, S. (1993) Discovery of the discharge process: a study of patient discharge from a care unit for elderly people. *Journal of Advanced Nursing*, **18**, 1288–96.

Jewell, S. (1994) Patient participation: what does it mean to nurses? *Journal of Advanced Nursing*, **19**, 433–8.

Kelly, T.A. and O'Leary, M. (1992) *The Nursing Skill Mix in the District Nursing Service*, NHSME Value for Money Unit, HMSO, London.

Kitson, A. (1991) *Therapeutic Nursing and the Hospitalised Elderly*, Scutari Press, London.

McFarlane, J.K. and Castledine, G. (1982) *A Guide to the Practice of Nursing Using the Nursing Process*, Mosby, St Louis.

Mackenzie, A. (1989) *Key Issues in District Nursing. Paper 1. The District Nurse Within the Community Context*, District Nurse Association, London.

Manthey, M. (1980) A theoretical framework for primary nursing. *Journal of Nursing Administration*, **10**(6), 54–6.

Manthey, M. (1988) Can primary nursing survive? *American Journal of Nursing*, **8**(5), 644–7.

Marriner, A. (1983) *The Nursing Process: A Scientific Approach to Nursing Care*, 3rd edn, Mosby, St Louis.

Maslow, A.H. (1943) A theory of human motivation. *Psychological Review*, **50**, 370–89.

Norton, D. (1965) Nursing in geriatrics. *Gerontologia Clinica*, **7**, 57–60.

Norton, D. (1977) Geriatric nursing – what it is and what it is not. *Nursing Times*, **73**, 1622–3.

Norton, D., McLaren, R. and Exton-Smith, A.N. (1962) *An Investigation of Geriatric Nursing Problems in Hospital*, National Corporation for the Care of Old People, London, reprinted 1976 by Churchill Livingstone.

Orem, D. (1980) *Nursing – Concepts of Practice*, 2nd edn, McGraw Hill, New York.

Prophit, P. (1980) *Documentation of the Nursing Process: The Reasons for Records*, Working Group on the documentation of the nursing process, World Health Organization, Copenhagen.

Roper, N., Logan, W. and Tierney, A. (1985) *The Elements of Nursing*, 2nd edn, Churchill Livingstone, Edinburgh.

Roy, C. (1976) *Introduction to Nursing: An Adaption Model*. Prentice Hall, Old Tappan, New Jersey.

Royal College of Nursing (1991) *The Role of the Nurse in Rehabilitation of Elderly People*, Scutari Press, London.

Rudd, T. (1954) *The Nursing of the Elderly Sick. A Practical Handbook for Geriatric Nursing*, Faber, London.

Sheppard, B. (1994) Patient's views of rehabilitation. *Nursing Standard*, **9**(10), 27–30.

Townsend, P. (1986) Ageism and social policy, in *Ageing and Social Policy. A Critical Assessment* (eds C. Phillipson and A. Walker) Gower Publishing, Aldershot.

Waters, K. (1986) The role of nursing in rehabilitation. *CARE – Science and Practice*, **5**(3), 17–21.

Wright, S. (1990) *My Patient, My Nurse*, Scutari Press, London.

FURTHER READING

Department of Health (1991) *The Patient's Charter*, Department of Health, London.
United Kingdom Central Council for Nursing, Midwifery and Health Visiting (1992) *Code of Professional Conduct*, UKCC, London.

Feet and footwear of older people   11

Olwen Finlay and Colin Fullerton

INTRODUCTION

In older people, independence can be hindered or limited by painful feet and unsuitable footwear and these can have an indirect but substantial effect on health and lifestyle. Mobility, essential to the quality of life and often the key to independent living, can be hindered by foot problems that are not felt to be important enough for the older person, family or formal carers to seek advice or treatment. Many people accept foot problems as an inescapable accompaniment of ageing and often do not realize that change has occurred, due to its insidious or longstanding nature (Neale, Boyd and Whiting, 1989). Other patients may be embarrassed by the shape of their feet, and some patients may forget to complain, as other pathologies possibly predominate in their mind. General practitioners may neglect assessment of the foot, as such pathologies are not immediately life threatening. The feet are usually covered with slippers or some form of footwear, thereby not alerting other members of the team to their state. The importance of assessing foot health and footwear needs, and having an efficient method of supplying footwear where needed, is essential if the impact of a proactive and timely rehabilitation programme is to be achieved (Finlay, 1995). A general assessment of the older person by any member of the team is incomplete without including the feet and footwear, and knowledge is needed of what to look for, how to manage it, and what to refer on.

INITIAL ASSESSMENT OF THE FEET

A brief assessment of the feet by any team member can quickly determine if referral is required for further management. Many older people equate their age and priority status with a 'right' to chiropody for the remainder of their lives, and although it is estimated that 50% of older people require foot health services (Clarke, 1969), others require more basic care. The key is ensuring that needs are met appropriately, and carers' access to a chiropodist for advice, training and assessment of the patient, where warranted, is essential. Foot health management covers basic foot care, chiropody and surgical podiatry. All levels are complemented by the availability of suitable footwear and a team approach.

BASIC FOOT CARE

Basic foot care is part of personal care. At the most rudimentary level it involves foot washing, drying and nail cutting. These tasks are generally undertaken by the older person or their carer as part of general care. Carers may be relatives, home carers, district nurses or carers in residential care homes and nursing homes. Adequate arrangements for the initial and continuing training of carers in basic foot care provision should be undertaken by state registered chiropodists (Department of Health, 1994). However, for those patients with pathological foot conditions and/or a systemic disorder such as diabetes or peripheral vascular disease, there may be a requirement for chiropody, in conjunction with ongoing self care.

Where older people cannot continue with their own uncomplicated self care, voluntary organizations in some areas provide a nail cutting service. Age Concern (England) has liaised with The Society of Chiropodists and Podiatrists to produce ethically based guidelines on simple nail cutting for the Age Concern (England) volunteers (Society of Chiropody and Age Concern, 1995). This includes state registered chiropodist involvement in training of volunteers, initial and annual assessment and provision of care for 'at risk' patients. Training for both informal and formal carers is equally important, if those at most risk are to be identified for chiropody, and others have appropriate self care or help from their carers.

Whatever foot care programme is indicated from the assessment, foot health education should be included. For older people this should include the basic principles of routine foot care and information on when and how to obtain NHS foot care in their locality. Additional information on the standards and qualifications of practising chiropodists and podiatrists should be clearly outlined.

CHIROPODY

Chiropody provides a comprehensive foot health service for conditions affecting the foot and lower limbs. State registered chiropodists undertake a 3–4 year state-approved training course and are eligible for work in the NHS. Non-registered chiropodists can undertake a variety of courses and are not eligible for work in the NHS. Foot care assistants provide simple foot care, under the supervision of a chiropodist, for patients who have previously been examined by a state registered chiropodist.

At the initial consultation between patient and chiropodist a detailed subjective account of the patient's concerns must be recorded. These may range from basic foot care problems to more complex foot pathologies related to systemic disease. A detailed objective examination by the chiropodist should include toenails, skin, the alignment of toes, the patient's medical history (to discount systemic disease, which may indirectly affect the feet), medication (e.g. steroids), observation of the patient's gait, examination of the patient's foot for biomechanical imbalances, assessment of the patient's neurological and vascular status, and footwear. The use of further laboratory analysis and imaging techniques may be necessary to obtain an accurate insight into the patient's pathology.

A diagnosis is made and a suitable programme of foot care can be tailored to the patient's needs. Before any attempt is made to implement this programme, the findings from the examination must be discussed with the patient. It is important that the patient or carer be given as much information as possible about the patient's foot health, in the form of verbal and written explanations. The chiropodist must talk to the patient or carer about the proposed treatment plan, which may or may not include chiropody treatment. Without compliance of the patient or carer, attempting to implement a treatment programme is doomed to failure.

After the treatment plan is completed, the outcome must be evaluation by the chiropodist and patient/carer. A further episode of care may be implemented if required. As practitioners may not have instant cures for pathologies within the ageing foot, the major aims should be to provide comfort, prevent complications, encourage walking, reduce pain and improve healing.

The following section covers problems commonly seen in the older foot, their causes, management by informal or formal carers and indications for referral to chiropody.

TOENAIL DISORDERS

Toenail disorders are common in older people (Helfand, 1981). The common causes of toenail pain are:

- ingrown toenails;
- abnormally thickened nails;
- infection of the nail bed;
- a bony nodule under the nail bed (exostosis);
- a corn underneath the nail;
- systemic disease associated with ageing.

Ingrown toenails result in symptoms ranging from mild discomfort to acute pain, and can cause infection and abscess formation where referral to the chiropodist is advised for conservative or surgical treatment, and to the general practitioner for antibiotics.

Thickening of the toenail occurs following some permanent damage to the nail matrix caused by trauma, back pressure from footwear, certain fungal nail infections or systemic nail conditions such as psoriasis. In this condition the nail plate is abnormally thickened with dark brownish discoloration. Overlying pressure from footwear causes pain and discomfort to the underlying nail bed. The excessive thickness makes nail cutting difficult. Using a nail drill, the chiropodist can reduce the thickness of the nail painlessly. As the damage is irreversible, regular treatment by the chiropodist will be necessary, otherwise neglect may result in a 'ram's horn' nail, affecting mobility (Figure 11.1).

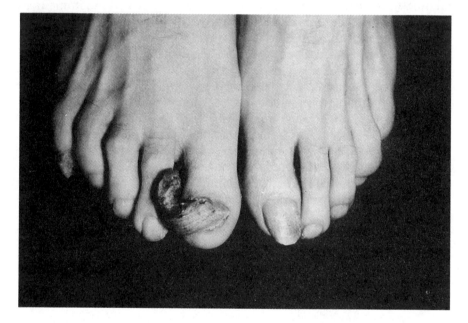

Figure 11.1 Ram's horn nail.

A **fungal infection** of the nail plate is commonly seen in the elderly patient, causing the nail plate to thicken with a yellow/brown discoloration (Beaven, 1984). Routine care by the chiropodist with the nail nippers and a nail drill will keep these nails reduced in bulk and pain free, or they may require systemic treatment from the general practitioner.

Infection of the soft tissues adjacent to the nail plate, such as paronychia, can spread to the underlying bone, especially in the presence of diabetes mellitus and vascular insufficiency. This requires immediate treatment with systemic antibiotics and local drainage of the wound. with suitable sterile dressings. Reduction of trauma to the area can be obtained by wearing modified footwear.

A **bony exostosis** occurs under the nail plate near its distal aspect. Surgery may reduce discomfort.

A **subungual corn** is located under the nail plate. Management consists of partial removal of the toenail and the underlying corn, with measures to modify footwear to remove pressure from the toe.

Systemic disease, such as psoriasis, can cause damage to the nail structure. The nail becomes thickened, pitted, crumbly and discolored. Regular treatment is required by the chiropodist to reduce the thickness of the nail.

LESSER TOE DEFORMITIES

Lesser toe deformities are often described as hammer, claw, retracted or mallet toes (Figure 11.2). Causes include muscle imbalance, due to wasting of the distal intrinsic muscles, and improperly fitting footwear, or an excessively long toe, which is traumatized by footwear. As toe deformities require increased depth within the toe box of the shoe, toes are often crushed, risking the formation of corns and calluses.

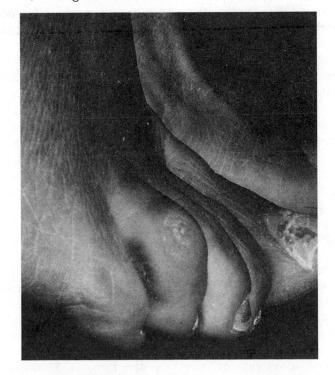

Figure 11.2 Lesser toe deformities.

Corns and calluses are a reaction of the skin to compressive, shearing and tensile stresses or unyielding footwear. A callus is a diffuse hypertrophy of the stratum corneum caused by compression and shearing stress. A corn is a circumscribed area of callus that has become increasingly compacted at the point of pressure from the shoe. The deepest portion of the corn impinges on the sensory nerve endings, resulting in pain. As corn and callus are derived from the stratum corneum, this can be removed painlessly, without bleeding. Shields can be fabricated out of wool felt or silicone material to reduce pressure on the affected toe. However, shields can only be comfortably worn if there is adequate accommodation within the shoe.

Patients and their carers often attempt self treatment of corns and callus. This may involve unsterile cutting instruments and proprietary corn cures, which often contain salicylic acid. In older patients with poor peripheral blood flow, incorrectly used home treatments may result in soft tissue infections and unnecessary chemical burns to the skin. Referral to the chiropodist would be appropriate.

FOREFOOT DISORDERS

Forefoot disorders are often the end result of primary biomechanical defects of the lower limb or foot which are compounded by contributory factors such as ill-fitting footwear or previous occupational stresses (Boyd, 1993).

The primary biomechanical defects are caused by postural deformities and structural malalignments of the lower limb and foot. The common defects are genu valgum (knock knees) or genu varum, which compound mobility problems. These structural defects should be treated at an earlier stage, before the sequelae of forefoot deformities become irreversible and chronic in nature. Where appropriate, inside heel wedges or casted functional orthoses can be fabricated to enhance foot function. However, in the aged foot, the chronic outcomes of biomechanical defects are clinically apparent as hallux valgus (Figure 11.3), hallux rigidus (rigid first metatarsophalangeal joint), bunionette deformity of the fifth metatarsophalangeal joint, plantarflexed or dorsiflexed first and fifth metatarsals and Morton's neuroma.

Morton's neuroma is essentially a degenerative process of the plantar digital nerve, which becomes irritated or crushed by the metatarsal heads. The symptoms vary in severity from an occasional 'pins and needles' sensation to a sudden and acute pain around the metatarsal heads, which brings the sufferer to a halt. Shoes that unduly constrict the forefoot may precipitate or worsen the pain, and relief is often obtained by removing the shoe and massaging or squeezing the forefoot. Management can involve digital and metatarsal padding to re-align the metatarsal bones

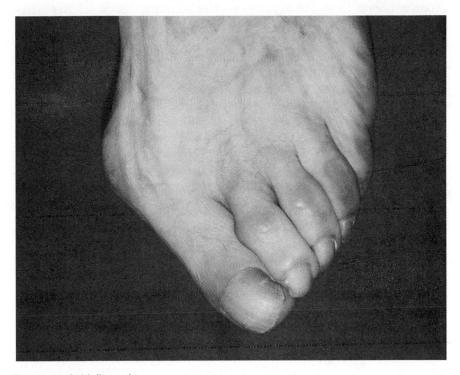

Figure 11.3 Hallux valgus.

and remove pressure from the digital nerve. If there is no success with conservative treatment, referral would be required for surgical resection of the offending digital nerve.

Functional orthoses are utilized to correct the biomechanical imbalances of the foot and softer material. Although these provide less correction, they are better tolerated by the older patient.

MID-FOOT DISORDERS

The three most common mid-foot disorders are ganglion formation, osteoarthritis of the first metatarsocuneiform joint and tenosynovitis.

A **ganglion** is a fluid-filled cyst usually derived from a tendon sheath or a joint capsule. The swelling can be readily manipulated from one part of the cyst to another. This, together with the very soft character of the swelling, distinguishes it from a bursa. Ganglia are often asymptomatic and may be left alone.

Osteoarthritis, resulting from the effects of wear and tear on the mid-foot joints, affects foot function. Management of this problem includes modification of footwear, to allow greater accommodation for the osteophytic outgrowths. Alternatively, the osteophytic lipping may be removed surgically.

Tenosynovitis may affect the tendon sheaths anterior to the ankle. The symptoms are swelling and pain along the tendon sheath, stiffness and crepitus on movement. The tendons stand out from the dorsum of the toe and are liable to be continually irritated by the crease in the upper of the shoe. A small hard corn may first develop, and removal may expose a sinus leading to the tendon. An infection may occur through the sinus. Management involves removal of pressure by appropriate pressure dispersion pads, with regular saline soaks if infection occurs, and referral to the patient's general practitioner for antibiotics if infection is a recurring problem.

HEEL DISORDERS

Heel disorders can be caused by:

- lipoatrophy
- plantar fasciitis
- calcaneal bursitis
- seronegative arthropathy
- marginal heel callus with fissures.

Some of the above disorders can be difficult to diagnose and treat, the thickness of the heel pad masking the clinical signs of inflammation.

Lipoatrophy cannot be classed as a disorder, but with the ageing process the thickness of the heel pad reduces. The property of shock absorption is reduced and the transmission of pressure is directed onto the underlying heel bone, with resulting pain and a tendency to walk by putting as little weight on the heels as possible, risking instability. Heel cushions and soft-soled footwear will help reduce the pain.

Plantar fasciitis is an inflammatory lesion at the junction between the plantar aponeurosis and the calcaneum. This common heel condition may be associated with a heel spur. Localized pain occurs first thing in the morning or after a period of rest. Management includes reducing the tensile stress on this attachment by the use of functional orthoses, the use of physical therapies to reduce the inflammatory response and, finally, steroid injection if other measures fail.

Posterior calcaneal bursitis is usually inflammation of subcutaneous bursa overlying the Achilles tendon insertion. Tenderness will be palpable directly over the calcaneus at the tendon insertion. A noticeable bursal thickening may be present over the bony prominence lateral to the tendon attachment. Footwear with a soft heel counter or soft cushion material adhering to the inside of the heel counter may reduce pressure on the overlying skin.

Marginal heel callus with fissures commonly occurs in the elderly population. This is associated with dry skin, obesity and wearing open-heeled footwear. As a result, the marginal heel skin is pinched against the rim of the sandal and callus is then formed. If the skin is excessively dry, the skin will split to form fissures as a result of the tensile and shearing forces that occur around the heel margins. Treatment consists of skin moisturizing lotions and advice on footwear such as avoidance of an open heel.

Plantar heel pain is also caused by systemic pathology such as seronegative arthropathy. Pain occurs at the attachment of ligaments and tendons to the underlying bone. A characteristic fluffy heel spur occurs at the junction of the plantar aponeurosis and the calcaneum (Jacoby, 1991).

WHOLE FOOT DISORDERS

The incidence of pes cavus (high arched foot) and pes planus (flatfoot) are not linked with the ageing foot. However, the ageing skin predisposes to the formation of corn and callus in areas of excessive pressure. The main disorders are:

- those of the skin
- systemic disease
- infections and ulceration
- malignancy.

SKIN DISORDERS OF THE FOOT

Tinea pedis is a fungal infection that commonly presents between the toes or in the area of the longitudinal arch. Symptoms include erythema and pruritis. The use of topical anti-fungal agents and footwear that permits ventilation (sandals) is the first line of action. Occlusive footwear made from synthetic substances is to be avoided. For the more acute and resistant fungal infections, referral to the general practitioner for systemic anti-fungal agents is necessary, but results in the elderly are disappointing, due to the decreased vascular supply inhibiting the systemic response.

The incidence of **verrucae** is relatively low in the elderly population compared to the teenage population, but they are very resistant to treatment. If the verruca is giving no pain, the lesion can be left untreated; if painful, proprietary lotions can be used with care.

Dry skin is a problem for a large proportion of older people, and contributes to the development of fissures, which can lead to infection. The frequent use of skin emollients help keep the skin soft by preventing moisture loss.

FOOT CONDITIONS AS RESIDUALS OF SYSTEMIC DISEASE

Diabetes mellitus is known to be responsible for multiple foot complications and, sometimes, foot symptoms will lead to the detection of the disease, the incidence of which increases with age. Foot manifestations often result from the sequelae of peripheral neuropathy and vascular pathology (Davidson, 1991).

Peripheral neuropathy consists of one or all three of the following components: sensory, autonomic and motor neuropathy, which together have the potential to put the foot at major risk.

Sensory neuropathy makes the patient unaware of minor abrasions to the foot and the risk of pressure-related ulceration. With **motor neuropathy**, the most distal muscles of the foot no longer obtain innervation, which results in clawing of the toes. This increases the weight-bearing pressures underneath the metatarsal heads. With **autonomic neuropathy**, the controlling innervation to the blood vessel wall is absent or reduced and the secretions of the sebaceous and sweat glands are reduced.

Vascular pathology associated with diabetes consists of microangiopathy (involving arteriolar vessels of the skin) and macroangiopathy (involving the medium- and large-sized arteries of the lower limb). Both conditions reduce the lumen of the vessel and therefore produce a reduced blood flow to the foot. The clinical effects are diminished or absent foot pulses, an increased risk of infection and possible ulceration with gangrene as a result. Systemic antibiotics are ineffective in these cases, as the blood supply is unable to distribute the drug to the target site. Neuropathic ulcers in elderly diabetics can be resistant to treatment. Management involves rest, systemic antibiotics to control infection, removal of dead tissue in ulcerated sites and measures to redistribute weight-bearing pressures. Many patients with an ulcerated lesion can be managed by conservative means for long periods of time. Once the ulcer is healed, prevention of future ulceration is essential. Referral to the diabetic multidisciplinary team is essential for appropriate management (McInnes, 1994).

Osteoarthritis elsewhere in the body, together with chronic trauma, strain and obesity are reflected in the weight-bearing joints of the foot. A reduced range of joint motion, altered foot pressures and the laying down of additional bone surrounding the focus joint is manifested. With altered plantar pressure distribution, corn and callus may occur and this should be referred to the chiropodist for management.

Peripheral vascular insufficiency is present to varying degrees in the majority of older people (Helfand, 1981) accompanied by pain, coldness, pallor, paraesthesia, burning, atrophy of soft tissues, dry skin, loss of hair and absent foot pulses. The final result of severe arterial occlusion is gangrene. Where peripheral blood flow is compromised, any abrasion caused by routine foot care can have disastrous results. Referral to the general practitioner for vasodilator medication or referral to a vascular surgeon for assessment is necessary.

Gout may produce symptoms in any joint of the foot and should always be suspected where intense pain is present without trauma. The signs and symptoms include chronic painful and stiff joints, soft tissue tophi, deformity and functional impairment. Referral to the general practitioner for investigation is appropriate. If the diagnosis is confirmed, systemic medication is required to control the metabolic imbalance.

Rheumatoid arthritis is accompanied in its later stages by exacerbation of pain, joint swelling, stiffness, muscle wasting and marked deformity of the feet. Management involves basic foot care, skilled management of foot ulceration and pressure dispersion pads for the sole of the foot. Referral for appropriate footwear is essential. If temporary footwear is required, it is essential that the design chosen alleviates pressure on the forefoot joints (Kinsman, 1980; Harrison, 1984)

Foot infection is a serious complication for the older person. It may be related to systemic disease or result from poor self care of a local foot problem. Residual deformities of earlier conditions, together with the ageing process, provide an excellent medium for the development of foot infections. Foot infections are the most common precipitant of amputation. Common causes of foot infections are:

- any trauma that causes a break in the skin;
- ill-fitting footwear and lack of self care;
- dryness of the skin, due to the ageing process;
- metabolic diseases such as diabetes mellitus combined with peripheral vascular disease.

Management involves removal of the exciting cause, saline foot soaks and referral to the general practitioner for systemic antibiotics, and ultimate hospitalization if systemic disease is uncontrolled.

Ulcerative lesions in the ageing foot are the result of localized pressure due to biomechanical dysfunction and are usually associated with metabolic disease such as diabetes mellitus or peripheral vascular insufficiency. Ulcers in the diabetic patient are usually painless, but an ischaemic ulcer is very painful and usually exhibits early local necrosis. Referral to the appropriate clinical department is essential. When healing occurs, all steps must be taken to prevent re-occurrence.

Malignancy affecting the foot is rare, but prompt referral to the general practitioner is essential for all suspicious new growths. The most common growths are melanoma and basal cell tumours (French, 1993). Melanomas often result from the conversion of benign moles to a malignant state. Any mole that increases in size, changes colour with serous fluid exuding from the surface should be treated with suspicion and immediately referred for a specialist opinion. Occasionally a melanoma can occur under the nail plate. As it gets bigger, the nail plate is eroded away, to give an appearance of subungual ulceration.

SURGICAL PODIATRY

Where foot problems cannot be fully met by conservative methods, surgery may be needed. Until recently this would have been undertaken by an orthopaedic surgeon, but a growing number of chiropodists are qualifying as surgical podiatrists, and are able to undertake some of this work (Department of Health, 1994).

As can be seen from the above, awareness and prevention of problems, particularly through suitable footwear, can go a long way to ensuring that feet are fit to facilitate rehabilitation.

FOOTWEAR

The footwear needs of older people may be quite simple and basic, but some patients with severely disordered feet require semi-bespoke or made-to-measure shoes (Pratts, 1989). Uncomfortable shoes can reduce their wearer's pleasure more than any other item of clothing and painful feet discourage mobility.

The majority of older people can have their needs met satisfactorily from the commercial market. The frail elderly may need additional help with supply and fitment. The commercial market should be properly researched before more expensive prescribed footwear is pursued. If feet are badly misshapen, then referral to an orthotist (surgical fitter) for appropriate footwear may be necessary to prevent the problems described in the first section of this chapter.

The aim is to maintain pain-free mobility for the patient, sustain safety and independence and thus enhance the quality of life. Footwear management should be considered as a treatment technique that can be employed to maintain or restore mobility. Although various healthcare professionals can provide this service, physiotherapists are in a unique position to assess the patient's total mobility needs. When this can be in conjunction with a chiropodist, the outcome can be further enhanced.

PRACTICAL PROBLEMS IN FOOTWEAR PROVISION: THE EXPERIENCE IN A PHYSIOTHERAPY DEPARTMENT

When many elderly people are admitted to hospital, footwear is often found to be unsuitable, non-existent, or potentially dangerous (Finlay, 1987). With an increasing ageing population, this problem is rising (Finlay, 1995).

PURPOSE OF SCREENING

The principal role of the physiotherapist in elderly care is to maximize the physical function of individual patients, with mobility and gait analysis being part of the treatment process. Treatment should be carried out in a safe environment. As footwear is part of that environment (Woollacott, Shumway-Cook and Nashner, 1982), therapists have a responsibility to advise, supply and if necessary, help with fitment, ensuring the product supplied maximizes function, permits normal foot movement and encourages locomotion. As it is not uncommon for patients to be admitted with ill-fitting shoes (Kwok, 1994), it is imperative that footwear be assessed and if necessary provided quickly to ensure that the physiotherapy rehabilitation programme is not adversely affected and to prevent any inappropriate bed usage (Finlay, 1994).

Footwear management requires a wide range of skills and knowledge. Often management can be very difficult, necessitating accurate information from the assessment process before advice can be given on shoe fitment. Gait analysis is the science and art of correlating clinical findings with objectively quantified biomechanical parameters that present during posture and locomotion.

If the patient's own footwear does not fulfil the criteria for safety (Finlay, 1987), then verbal and written advice should be provided for the patient and carer (if appropriate) and if possible help with fitment and supply, as this can enhance the impact of physiotherapy. An example of such a scheme is shown in Figure 11.4.

OBJECTIVES OF A FOOTWEAR SCHEME

1. To identify those people with footwear unsuited to their needs and provide explanation and advice;
2. To provide an economical, well fitting shoe, suited to individual need;
3. To organize an effective service that would be 'need' responsive, assisting the wearer to stand, balance and move (if possible) in comfort and safety;
4. To assist the elderly (especially the frail elderly) to cope with purchasing a correct product in a complex marketplace;
5. To reduce waiting time for patients to obtain footwear;
6. To provide sufficient information to help the patient and carer to reach an informed decision, thus improving patient satisfaction;
7. To refer on for specialist provision where needs cannot be met through the commercial market or in house adaptation service;
8. To increase environmental safety, by decreasing the number of older people who are at risk by wearing unsafe shoes (Figure 11.5).

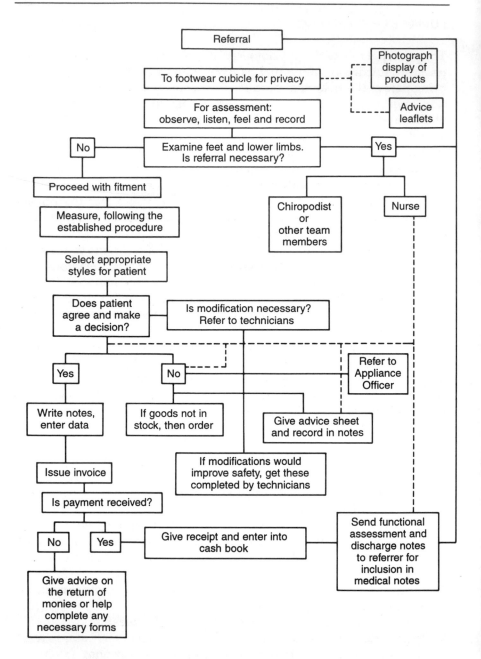

Figure 11.4 Flow chart showing standardized procedure for footware supply in a physiotherapy department.

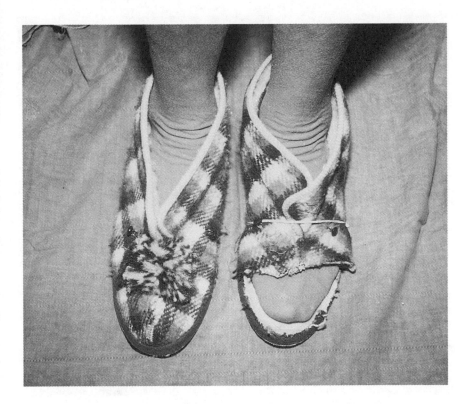

Figure 11.5 An example of unsafe shoes.

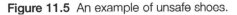

Footwear is of real, but often unrecognized, psychological importance to the wearer. Shoes, which are always visible, can reflect self image and identity, and adults who have to wear special footwear and can no longer wear preferred styles may lose those important symbols of image and identify. They may also for the first time be confronted with a visible symbol of their disability (Disabled Living Foundation, 1990).

One of the problems associated with this area of care is the complexity of the variables, such as weight, age, range of joint movement, sex and cadence (length of stride), and it is often a complex issue to cater for individual need (Finlay, 1995). Often the elderly person's foot is unique (Figure 11.6).

Little account may be taken in retail outlets of the differences in foot structure of minority groups, the typical slender Asian and broad African foot having to be accommodated in a European mould. There are obvious foot health and general safety issues, and such poor fitment may lead to 'treading down' of the back of the shoe, with a subsequent effect on mobility, as well as on the skin of the heel.

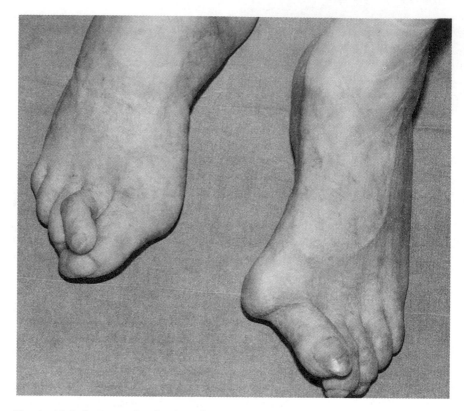

Figure 11.6 An example of unique feet.

The physiotherapist must have a sound knowledge of the anatomy of the foot and lower limb and have the ability to analyse problems in gait with a clear understanding of the interplay between footwear, walking and balance (Dunne *et al.*, 1993) in patients of all ages.

AIMS FOR CONSERVATIVE FOOT MANAGEMENT

1. Relieve pain, providing comfort;
2. Ensure the foot is as functional as possible;
3. Maintain pain-free movements;
4. Compensate for any disturbance of normal weight bearing.

The initial examination is important, including history, feel, measurement, range of movement as well as observation. It is important to note that hindfoot function should always be observed by standing behind the person being assessed. Records should include essential information relating to calluses, circulation, skin changes and gait problems and examination of regularly worn footwear – often a story in themselves.

Excessive wear on the heels may indicate long periods of sitting with repetitive heel shuffling, while wear on the anterior and lateral border of the shoe may indicate a drop foot before it is visible to the eye. Excessive wear on either the medial or lateral borders of the heel will reflect uneven alignment of weight or possibly instability. Misshapen uppers often indicate the presence of bunions and potential areas of excessive friction. Pristine soles may indicate that these are not the shoes normally used but 'Sunday best', and the regular shoes must be requested.

EFFECT OF SHOE STYLE ON GAIT

Slip-on shoes or slippers will increase the tendency to shuffle; shiny or plastic soles will produce a fearful, small-step gait; narrow styles will inhibit normal foot movement, reducing normal toe function and preventing normal toe 'push off', affecting gait pattern and weight transference. Obese patients will find wedge heeled shoes more supportive than a 'waisted' shoe and the uppers will retain their shape longer. Narrow tapering heels will increase instability. Thick mid-soles will increase the tendency to fall in older people, as these shoes tend to have an 'edge effect', whereby they resist compression less at their edges than in the centre, resulting in destabilization (Robbins, Gouw and McClaran, 1992). Increased softness probably worsens foot position awareness and impairs stability (Robbins, Gouw and McClaran, 1995). More research into the design of footwear for 60-year-olds and above would be useful (Nigg and Skleryk, 1988), because if ill fitting shoes slow the speed of movement then this increases the vulnerability of elderly people during such activities as crossing roads (Finlay, 1993; Hoxie and Rubenstein, 1994).

The importance of patient involvement in the decision-making process and of encouraging them to take some responsibility for their own health cannot be over-stressed, as there is a reported waste of £2 000 000 per annum within the NHS from the provision of unacceptable footwear (Platts, 1989).

STANDARDS FOR A QUALITY FOOTWEAR SERVICE

1. All patients are screened in privacy by a therapist skilled in gait analysis and shoe fitment.
2. Accurate measurements are recorded in individual notes.
3. Adequate information is provided, so that all patients understand the importance of safe footwear and the dangers of ignoring advice.
4. If a change is required, explanation is provided for the need for the change.
5. Patients are involved in the decision-making process.

It is not unreasonable to expect the majority of patients to be supplied **within three working days** of referral (Finlay, 1995), if the hospital operates an 'off the shelf' service. Under national contracts, bespoke footwear should be delivered within six weeks (Michaelson, 1989).

MEASUREMENTS TO BE TAKEN DURING AN ASSESSMENT

- Length, using a British standard foot gauge;
- Footprints taken in standing, if possible, or better during locomotion and using underplantar pressure technology;
- Metatarsal depth, using thermoplastic bridges;
- Angle at first metatarsophalangeal joint;
- Heel girth (especially important when swelling is a problem).

This will provide the necessary information to indicate the most appropriate style for the individual.

The most common problems the physiotherapists would be likely to encounter are shown in Figure 11.7.

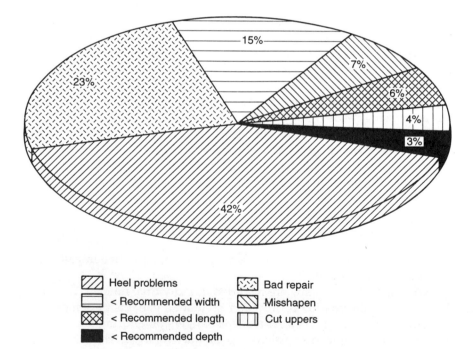

Figure 11.7 Common footwear problems seen on admission.

Problems	Alternatives/Solutions
Nail problems	Refer to the chiropodist. Possibly deep footwear required.
Corn and callosities	Refer to the chiropodist. Supply extra deep footwear with sufficient room in the toe box to prevent any undue pressure or friction. A poron tongue pad helps hold the foot back into the heel cup, and reduces the pressure on the forefoot.
Claw or hammer toes	Provide extra deep shoes, to prevent any undue pressure or friction on the forefoot.
Mild swelling	Action will depend on degree of swelling; mild pitting may only require extra wide/deep shoes. Graduated pressure stockings may be helpful.
Gross swelling	Tweed covered plastazote shoes can be used as a short-term solution. Other modalities such as intermittent pressure therapy and graduated pressure support stockings may run concurrently. Encourage increased mobility. Ankle and foot exercises may be required.
Hallux valgus	Extra deep footwear. Footwear may require modification to increase area in contact with the ground. Gait re-education.
Ulcers and circulatory conditions	Ensure the interior of the shoe is as smooth as a velvet glove. Provide insoles that assist in re-distribution of the weight if necessary. Ensure information leaflets are supplied.
Real leg shortening	A raise should be applied, tapered towards the toe, to facilitate easier swing-through during locomotion. The raise height can usually be reduced by 0.5 inch (8 mm) of the shortening differential.
Apparent leg shortening	No modification usually required.
Partial amputation of the foot	A shoe filler made from poron and plastazote can be moulded to fill the vacant space. Supply odd size shoes.
Complex foot deformities	Refer to the orthotist. Refer to chiropodist if required.

SOME BENCHMARKS FROM THE MEASUREMENTS REGARDING THE STYLE MOST LIKELY TO MEET THE PATIENT'S NEEDS

- Width of footprints at level of the first metatarsophalangeal joint.
  - >9.5 cm (ladies) will be accommodated by most commercial products.
  - >9.5 cm and <10.5 cm will require more expensive wider and deeper styles, often difficult to obtain in the high street, but available from specialist mail order suppliers or from medical orthopaedic footwear suppliers.
  - >10.5 cm are frequently unavailable, and will most probably require orthopaedic footwear. Vinyl/tweed products made in physiotherapy or chiropody departments can provide a satisfactory short-term measure. Choice will be governed by lifestyle.
- Depth
  The thermoplastic bridges are used to measure depth at the forefoot, angled from the first metatarsophalangeal joint to the fifth.
  - <3.5 cm will usually find sufficient space at the toe box in a commercial shoe.
  - >3.5 cm and <4.5 cm will require a deeper than average shoe, again not easily available in the marketplace.
  - >4.5 cm and <5.25 cm will require the semi-bespoke range with an extra deep toe box, and this is usually manufactured in an extra-wide width.
  - >5.25 cm will require orthopaedic or bespoke footwear, with approximately an eight-week delivery period. It is necessary in the short term to provide either vinyl or tweed, which can be cast and produced in less than three days.

THE SHOE PROVIDED

No single shoe suits the majority of people, but lightweight shoes are essential. The fastenings must be adequate and hold the foot well back into the shoe; either laces or Velcro are satisfactory and the latter is useful for those patients who have lost fine finger movements. Occupational therapy should be sought when finger movements are limited and fastenings need further adaptation.

Non-skid soles are essential, the only exception being Parkinsonian patients, who may find occasionally that leather permits and provides a slippage that facilitates movement. Deeply cleated or highly ridged soles are best avoided, as these tend to catch on certain types of carpet.

Although lifestyle may dictate the composition of the upper, little variation is acceptable in the heels. Low heels are vital (<3.5 cm), and the rheumatoid patient will benefit from an even lower heel height of 2.4 cm to reduce weight on the forefoot. Low heels provide greater stability and the width should be >5.5 cm, as this increases the area in contact with the ground and improves stability.

All footwear provided should allow the toes to move normally, without undue pressure or friction, and there should be at least 1.2 cm between the end of the longest toe and the inside of the shoes. Sufficient space should be provided in the toe box to prevent pressure or friction (Finlay, 1987).

Although patients may consider external appearance the most important factor, the interior should not be overlooked. For the diabetic patient or those with vulnerable skin, a smooth surface is vital. Canvas uppers often tend to have rough inside seams, and shoes with stitching often cause problems.

Patients with neuropathy or ischaemic problems require very soft leather uppers, increased depth, cushioning insoles and, when necessary, weight-distributing cradles with sinks and extra cushioning under high-pressure areas (Tovey and Platt, 1989).

UNDERPLANTAR PRESSURE TECHNOLOGY

The use of information technology now available to the therapist assists assessment by providing quantitative and qualitative information. The patient is required to walk over two plates, the position of which can be adjusted to accommodate individual stride length. A total of 2048 sensors record the underplantar pressure. The footprint data are displayed as coloured squares, each corresponding to the sensor on the plate. The colour of each area represents the pressure against time applied to that sensor; different colours correspond to different values, with the pressure values being displayed. The pressure is recorded in kg/cm^2. This system also provides colour dynamic footprints that can be obtained in two and three dimensions.

Figure 11.8 illustrates poor unsupportive slippers with poor heel counters, yet the gait analysis illustrated the extremely high pressure exerted at the heel on heel strike that required urgent remedial action. The means that it is invaluable to analyse gait scan by scan when modifications are prescribed, as the computer confirms problems often observed by the therapist and can provide a useful visual aid for patients.

MODIFICATIONS

The physiotherapist should be prepared to recommend footwear modifications, as almost 25% will require some type of modification to maximize function (Finlay, 1995). If underplantar pressure technology to provide scientific data is not available, then recommendations must be based on sound clinical judgement.

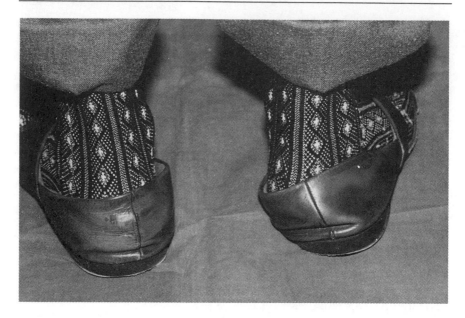

Figure 11.8 Unsupportive slippers with poor heel counters.

It is advantageous for the physiotherapist to have the skills to apply modifications on site. The cost effectiveness of this skill is soon appreciated by other team members, as it prevents unnecessary waste. If it is applied temporarily in the first instance and proves to be unacceptable or does not maximize function, more expensive permanent modifications should not be completed, but referral made for specialist advice.

WEDGES

A wedge may be applied to the sole or heel or both, depending on the amount of weight modification or re-alignment required. Ready made stick-on wedges of 3°, 4° or 5° are obtainable, but it is often more satisfactory to buff the wedge for individual need. The severity and type of deformity dictates the size, degree and position of the wedges. For example, 'back sliders' are often helped by wedges at the back of the heel, helping to prevent the backwards thrust, in the same way that a wedge at the front of the heel (1.5 cm to nothing) can help reduce antropulsion. Wedges placed on the medial sides of the soles and heels help minimize genu valgum or on the lateral side for genu varum. Post-cerebrovascular accident patients will occasionally require ankle re-alignment to prevent the ligaments being traumatized through abnormal stresses when weight bearing.

All wedges should be tried on a temporary basis before permanent application.

The amount of floor contact in the gait of a 96-year-old lady varied between 4.41 cm^2 and 45.51 cm^2 on the left foot and 2.24 cm^2 and 36.93 cm^2 on the right, in old canvas shoes (Figure 11.9). The area in ground contact improved significantly with appropriate footwear, with the area increasing to 21.63 – 68.28 cm^2 on the left foot and 2.61 – 77.58 cm^2 on the right foot, thus producing more stability.

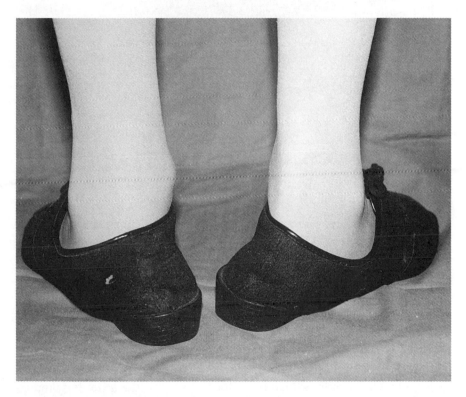

Figure 11.9 Variable amounts of floor contact by feet in these old canvas shoes.

FLOATS

Floats are provided to give added support by widening the heel and increasing the surface area in ground contact. Floats help prevent the breakdown of the heel counter when excess weight or abnormal stresses are present (Figure 11.10).

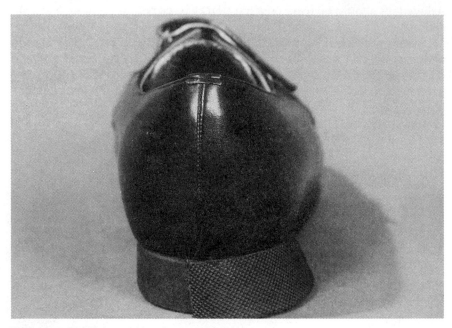

Figure 11.10 A shoe with a float on the heel.

TONGUE PADS

A tongue pad is a piece of poron (a closed cellular substance), rubber or orthopaedic felt stuck to the undersurface of the tongue of the shoe. These are invaluable if a foot tends to slip forward, causing unnecessary pressure on the forefront of the foot. The pad will help hold the foot back into the heel cup, permitting the forefront of the foot to move and function as normally as possible.

SUMMARY

Comfortable feet and safe footwear are essential for mobility and well being of older people. Whilst basic foot care is normally undertaken by people as part of their personal care, older people may need assistance. As feet do develop specific disorders in old age, a state registered chiropodist should provide advice following an assessment of the best foot care management programme. This may incorporate self care, chiropody or surgical podiatry. In all cases, footwear that is both safe and comfortable is an essential feature, and an example is given of an inexpensive but effective system to meet the needs of most older people unable to be catered for through retail outlets, but not requiring highly specialized bespoke footwear.

Shoes have been noted by many authors as a contributing factor to falls in older people (Dunne *et al.*, 1993). Substitution of a shoe that lessens risk of tripping may not prevent all falls, but it may represent an important intervention in the complex risk of falls. There is a need for increased awareness and more focus required on education of both the public and carers. It is hoped that this short description will illustrate how footwear influences and affects gait and how the physiotherapist with an understanding of the interplay between walking, balance and footwear can use this knowledge to maximize function in the older person.

TERMINOLOGY

Commercial footwear As bought in a high street store.

Extra wide footwear Difficult to obtain in the high street. Specialist mail order companies or an orthopaedic footwear supplier can supply these goods.

Semi-bespoke footwear Obtained from an orthopaedic footwear supplier. They generally weigh about 200 g/shoe (Herold and Palmer, 1992).

Bespoke footwear Tailor-made shoes only obtainable from a surgical/orthopaedic footwear supplier. They weigh about 800 g/shoe (Herold and Palmer, 1992).

Temporary plastazote/vinyl/tweed footwear Can be made in the physiotherapy department after casting with plaster of Paris bandages. A positive cast of the foot is obtained and the shoe is moulded. Simple equipment makes this product: e.g. scissors, leather knife, an oven for moulding and an electric drill with a buffer attachment.

Prescribed footwear Regulations in Great Britain state that 'Where the clinical needs of a patient can be met by the provision of a standard article, or such an article adapted, specially made appliances should not be supplied under the National Health Service' (National Health Service, 1985).

Chiropodist As mentioned in this chapter, this will be a state registered chiropodist.

Physiotherapist As mentioned in this chapter, this will be a state registered physiotherapist.

REFERENCES

Beaven, D.W. (1984) Fungal infections and onychomycosis, in *A Colour Atlas of the Nail*, Wolfe Medical Publications, London, pp. 82–9.

Boyd, P.M. (1993) The adult foot, in *Neale's Common Foot Disorders*, 4th edn (ed D.L. Lorimer), Churchill Livingstone, Edinburgh, p. 51.

Clarke, M. (1969) *Trouble with Feet*, G. Bell & Sons, London.

Davidson, M.B. (1991) An overview of diabetes mellitus, in *The High Risk Foot in Diabetes Mellitus* (ed R.G. Frykberg), Churchill Livingstone, New York, pp. 1–22.

Department of Health (1994) *Feet First*, Department of Health, London.

Disabled Living Foundation (1990) *Footwear – A Quality Issue*, Disabled Living Foundation, London.

Dunne, R.G., Bergman, A.B., Rogers, L.W. and Rivara, F.P. (1993) Elderly persons' attitudes towards footwear – a factor in preventing falls. *Public Health Reports*, **108**(2), 254.

Editorial (1990) Well shod. *Physiotherapy Journal*, **70**(9), 503.

Finlay, O. (1987) Footwear management in the elderly care programme. *Journal of the Society of Chiropodists*, **42**(5), 159–70.

Finlay, O. (1993) Exercise training and walking speeds in elderly woman following hip surgery, 'Beating the little green man'. *Physiotherapy Journal*, **70**(12), 845–9.

Finlay, O. (1994) *Stay Safe, Stay Steady*, post Malta conference report, World Confederation of Physical Therapists, London.

Finlay, O. (1995) The use of computers to assess problems associated with gait in elderly people. *Information Technology in Nursing*, **7.1**, 9–12.

French, G. (1993) The ageing foot, in *Neale's Common Foot Disorders*, 4th edn (ed D.L. Lorimer), Churchill Livingstone, p. 162.

Harrison, R.A. (1984) A simple pattern for plastozate boots. *Physiotherapy Journal*, **70**(6), 114–15.

Helfand, A.E. (1981) Primary foot care for the elderly, in *Clinical Podigeriatrics* (ed A.E. Helfand), Williams and Wilkins, Baltimore, p. 1–4.

Herold, D.C. and Palmer, R.G. (1992) Questionnaire study of the use of surgical shoes prescribed in a rheumatology outpatient clinic. *Journal of Rheumatology*, **19**(10), 1542–4.

Hoxie, R.E. and Rubenstein, L.Z. (1994) Are older people allowed enough time to cross intersections safely? *Journal of the American Geriatrics Society*, **42**, 241–4.

Jacoby, R.K. (1991) The painful foot in systemic disorders, in *The Foot and its Disorders* (ed L. Klenerman), Blackwell Scientific Publications, London, p. 131.

Kinsman, R. (1980) The do-it-yourself shoe. *Physiotherapy Journal*, **69**(9), 304–5.

Kwok, T. (1994) A survey of in-patient's footwear. *Care of the Elderly Journal*, **March**, 118.

McInnes, A.D. (1994) The role of the chiropodist, in *The Foot in Diabetes*, 2nd edn (eds A.J.H. Boulton, H. Connor, P.R. Cavanagh *et al.*), Wiley, Chichester, pp. 77–91.

Michaelson, P. (1989) Surgical footwear (letter). *British Medical Journal*, **299**, 1217.

National Health Service (1985) *General Arrangements for the Supply of Medical and Surgical Appliances and Orthopaedic Footwear in NHS patients*, NHS, Sheffield, pp. 2–3.

Neale, D., Boyd, P.M. and Whiting, M.F. (1989) The adult foot, in *Common Foot Disorders* (ed D. Neale and I.M. Adams), Churchill Livingstone, London, Melbourne and New York, p. 53.

Nigg, B.M. and Skleryk, B.N. (1988) Gait characteristics of the elderly. *Clinical Biomechanics*, **3**, 79–87.

Pratts, R.G.S. (1989) The NHS boot. *British Medical Journal*, **299**, 932–3.

Robbins, S., Gouw, G.J. and McClaran, J. (1992) Shoe sole thickness and hardness influence balance in older men. *Journal of the American Geriatrics Society*, **40**, 1089–94.

Robbins, S., Waked, E. and McClaren, J. (1995) Proprioception and stability: foot position awareness as a function of age and footwear. *Age and Ageing*, **24**, 67–72.

Society of Chiropody and Age Concern (1995) Voluntary nail-cutting guidelines. *Journal of British Podiatric Medicine*, **50**(5), 74.

Tovey, F.I. and Platt, H. (1989) Surgical footwear (letter). *British Medical Journal*, **299**, 1216.

Woollacott, M.H., Shumway-Cook, A. and Nashner, L.M. (1982) Postural reflexes and ageing, in *The Ageing Motor System* (eds J.A. Mortimer, F.J. Pirozzolo and G.J. Maletta), Praeger, New York, pp. 98–119.

The potential of social work in the rehabilitation of older people

12

Jill Manthorpe

The term social worker is often used in a broad sense to describe someone who works for a local authority social services department (England and Wales) or social work department (Scotland). The actual qualification of Diploma in Social Work (previously Certificate of Qualification in Social Work) defines a more restricted group of employees, but the majority of these are still based in local authorities. In this chapter, while not disregarding the often skilled and experienced work of other social services personnel, we focus on the work of qualified social workers in rehabilitation settings, acknowledging that many are in management positions, supervising others with more direct client contact. We look at the context of their work, key theories and values which underpin their practice and current concerns and contributions. By examining care management in particular, we explore some of the social work activities that impinge on the lives of older people and their helpers, professional or otherwise, in the area of rehabilitation and continuing care.

THE PROFESSION OF SOCIAL WORK

Social work as a profession has a number of differences from other professions engaged in rehabilitation work with older people. For example, strictly speaking it is not a profession, since members are not professionally autonomous, there is no General Social Work Council and the title is not protected. However, as Hugman (1991) has noted, social work is structurally independent from other professions and it sits comfortably with a range of other jobs in the classification of a 'caring profession', where members are committed to helping other people and where they express moral support and may give practical assistance. Nonetheless, the term 'caring' needs to be used cautiously, since as Clarke (1993) has observed, the history of social work is tied up with developments of industrialization and urbanization. These social changes have necessitated the growth of professional bureaucracies to respond to issues of social control as well as the care of social casualties.

The British social work profession has roots in a number of responses to social ills. In the area of rehabilitation the key origins lie in what we now term social work as practised by hospital almoners, who offered assistance to the sick poor but also ensured that a means test operated and hospital beds were cleared as rapidly as possible. The first hospital almoner, Mary Stewart, was appointed at the Royal Free Hospital in 1895. Beyond institutions, social work is also the consequence of voluntary and statutory relief of the poor, in the form of the Victorian philanthropic Charity Organisation Society and the Poor Law Board of Guardians (see Chapter 1).

Contemporary social work has come some way, and one might also argue full circle, in that despite calls for it to be a universal service (available to all), it is still mostly involved in the lives of poorer individuals. In spite of calls for it to be community focused, it still has substantial roles in institutionally provided care, such as in hospitals or prisons. Furthermore, in spite of calls for it to be engaged in liberationist or radical community development, much of social workers' time is spent implementing central government legislation on behalf of a local authority, who by employing social workers is able to carry out its legal obligations. Most social workers are employed by social services departments (England and Wales) or social work departments (Scotland). These are departments of local authorities who, through a committee structure, organize their activities. Each local authority may organize its services as it wishes to a large extent, but central government legislation or policy directive curtails its organizational autonomy.

Within the discussion of the professional context there are three points that might usefully be made in relation to the work force. These relate to gender, previous work history and training.

Most social workers are women, a fact that is particularly relevant in services for older people, where the majority are also women. However, as Grimwood and Popplestone (1993) have pointed out, women are concentrated in social work at the lower base of the job hierarchy. Although this probably comes as no surprise to women working in nursing, professions allied to medicine or medicine itself, gender is an important factor in relation to ageing experiences, including rehabilitation. Gender as a subject for debate among older people has begun to be explored and it frequently infuses discussions about informal care of older people by their relatives; as yet less information exists on the dynamics around gendered aspects of formal care and relationships between working women (see Langan and Day, 1992, for an exception).

The second point of relevance is to do with recruitment, in that many social workers come to this work with previous employment history. This is contrary to other trainee professionals (nurses, for example) who frequently arrive on vocational courses from full-time education. Whilst we are not able to predict the precise impact of alternative careers or work on professional activities, it is worth noting that social workers are increasingly likely to have had experience in residential or nursing home care and this may impact on their perceptions about rehabilitation, residential or nursing home life and older people (Manthorpe and Stanley, 1996). It has been a major feature of much residential care and nursing home provision that the role of rehabilitation has been unclear and little emphasized. Although many homes have taken over the role of convalescence facilities, the attitude of care assistants and others employed on a casual or part-time basis is unlikely to foster such positive attitudes without training and good role models (Lee-Treewick, 1994).

The third point is related to social work training. The qualification of Diploma in Social Work (DipSW) is awarded by the Central Council for Education and Training in Social Work. Students may undertake training for this qualification on a full-time or part-time basis, combining it with an undergraduate or postgraduate degree, or follow the Diploma course. The DipSW qualification is based on a broad concept of competence, which includes a variety of roles in caring, support, controlling and protecting people in need in relation to the wider community (for more details see CCETSW, 1991). Most social workers will have had academic input in areas such as law, psychology, social policy, sociology and community development. All will have had placements within agencies that assess their skills in individual and professional tasks such as assessment, service liaison and communication. The proposed reforms in social work education reflect the tensions between the shift to a competence-driven curriculum and the broader ethos of traditional higher education (Yelloly, 1995).

Currently social workers will have received wide-ranging and generic training, although most workers will have received more training in child care than in ageing or disability (Borsay, 1989). This is due to legal imperatives in the area of child protection and mental health together with employers' appreciation that problems in such publicly sensitive areas should be minimized by the more favourable allocation of trained staff. Training in areas such as ageing is given less priority (although the social work curriculum is relevant to the work of other professionals; see Biggs, 1993 and Ahmad-Aziz et al., 1992), but public sensitivities may force change. However, one of the findings from early community care research was that social workers often felt that they needed more medical 'nous' to help them understand the impact and consequences of medical conditions (Challis and Davies, 1986).

SOCIAL WORK WITH OLDER PEOPLE

Research among social workers is consistent in reporting that work with older people is unpopular. Some of the reasons affecting training and practice have been identified earlier. Moreover, fewer qualified social workers are appointed to work with older people, compared with child protection or mental health cases. Phillips (1992 p. 239) noted that, for many years, 'anyone working on the arena of eldercare was seen to be committing professional suicide', and that the new emphasis of the NHS and Community Care Act 1990 still questions whether social work is relevant to the process of providing help to older people. Work with this group highlights a central debate about the relationship between counselling (broadly defined) and services (see Pritchard and Brearley, 1982).

There may be more behind the ambivalence of many social workers than career motivation or the content of the work, for the needs of older people are rarely disputed. Biggs (1993) explores whether social workers hold stereotypes about the passivity of old people which are then mirrored by their own professional practices. This might account for the difficulty social workers can express in working creatively with older people and even in empathizing with their experiences.

The effects of other professional priorities and personal ambivalence have been studied in a variety of areas of social work. Phillipson and Biggs (1992) have suggested that they may help to explain the slow development of professional reaction to the issues of elder abuse. Challis and Davies (1986) found that inexperienced, untrained workers were often placed in positions in which residential care was the only option considered by both workers and older people. Marshall (1989) argued that, in relation to older people with dementia, protective legal structures are disregarded in a way that would not be deemed acceptable for other age groups.

WORKING TOGETHER EFFECTIVELY

Social work's relationship with professionals and workers from other agencies forms another key area in any exploration of social work practice and older people. It can be explored at three levels: between professionals, between organizations and at the national level. The first level is of interprofessional working and the relationships that exist between people employed in areas of work that are often concerned with improving the quality of life for older people, maximizing their independence and enabling them to function effectively in the face of sickness or disability.

Despite the apparent unanimity of aims, researchers have shown in practice that there are differences of approach and emphasis between professionals. Dalley (1989) reported that fundamental ideological differences existed between those involved in social work and those involved in healthcare. In her research she investigated professionals' views on whether the family or the state should be responsible for the care of old people. In general, she found that general practitioners inclined to the family model, nurses were at the midpoint in the spectrum and social workers were more in favour of state responsibility. Furthermore, Dalley observed that these divides might be exacerbated by 'tribal' allegiances, which separated professionals even when their ideological views were rather similar. It would not be surprising, therefore, to note that shared or agreed goals are difficult to establish at times (see also Chapters 4, 5 and 6). While individually professionals might argue that each acts in the best interests of the older patient or service user, it is helpful to appreciate how all are influenced by professional socialization. The current emphasis on empowerment as a key social work value, for example, means that many social workers are keen to establish a person's wishes and also to develop a context in which they are able to express their views, directly or indirectly, through advocacy (Dalrymple and Burke, 1995). As Dalley (1991) has added, differences in professionals' attitudes may inhibit collaboration, particularly when the force of circumstances combines with cultural or tribal allegiances. This implies that shared plans of care are rarely simple to deliver, if there are significant issues of risk or resources involved.

Perceived solutions to inter-professional rivalries and hostilities have been advanced in the area of joint training (Manthorpe and Hettiaratchy, 1993), multidisciplinary teams (such as primary care teams; Hutchinson and Gordon, 1992) and reflective practice. In the last, Pietroni (1992) has argued that difficulties in inter-professional communication may to some extent be based on discrete professional languages and their influences. The lack of knowledge of others' language, he has suggested, contributes to highly charged discussions rather than communication.

The second level of inter-professional working is often described as organizational collaboration or co-ordination. Most research has been fairly introspective and has concentrated on relationships between agencies such as social services departments and the NHS, education departments, the probation service and housing authorities. There is relatively little information on relationships with the voluntary sector (although see Davis Smith, Rochester and Hedley, 1995, for a good overview) or the commercial sector of care, despite their key roles in the provision of services to older people.

At this level the experiences of older people with both health and social care needs tends to typify organizational difficulties in working together. In a study of two health authorities, Wright, Ball and Coleman (1988) looked at services for older people with mental illness. They found that the hospital service, community health teams and social services departments tended to work in physical isolation, with little knowledge of each other and few formal links and laboured under frequent misapprehensions about the roles of other organizations.

There are a variety of structural explanations for such problems, such as the different forms of accountability and hierarchies between health and social services (Hunter, 1988). The impact of the NHS and Community Care Act 1990 changes, both separately and jointly, may well be towards increased joint planning, for example through the annual production of community care plans (Lewis, 1993).

These are part of a range of central government imperatives that aim to improve collaboration and are outlined in the White Paper *Caring for People* (Department of Health, 1989) and its voluminous guidance.

There is a third level of influence in working together to the benefit of older people and that is at the national or macro-level. It is at this level that priorities are established and principles adopted which translate into practice. A number of social work commentators have questioned whether central government has deliberately denied social work any role for the future in its continual references to 'the all embracing practitioner' (Cheetham, 1993, p. 157) and whether the future of local authorities is secure, with the introduction of the concept of enabling authorities, quasi-markets and joint commissioning (Nocon, 1994).

Most important it is at this level that decisions are made about the level of public expenditure and its priorities. As Tinker (1992) has noted, it is difficult to prove whether public expenditure reflects social services provision accurately, since financial costings are extremely blurred and complex. The continued poverty of large numbers of older people (one-third living at or below the poverty line; Walker, 1993) has immense impact on the work of social workers and other professionals working with older people. Social workers' impact at this level is marginal, especially since their own role, as we see in the next section, is now concentrated at the interpersonal level around assessment and care co-ordination.

ASSESSMENT AND CARE MANAGEMENT

No agreed definition of social work exists according to Taylor and Devine (1993), but theories point to the interaction between social worker and user as the important location of a problem-solving cycle. In many social services departments, organizational reforms following implementation of the NHS and Community Care Act 1990 have resulted in significant internal changes, relocating staff into quasi-purchasing and provider-type teams. Moreover, a number of authorities have also re-examined their provision of direct services, such as old people's residential homes, and domiciliary services, including home helps. Social workers may now find themselves in the purchasing arm

of a department, carrying out general assessments of adults and organizing care plans in the community. Alternatively, particularly in the
case of specialist staff such as Approved Social Workers (those who have
undertaken a post-qualifying course in mental health), some may be
working in specific locations carrying out legal responsibilities under
the Mental Health Act 1983.

The position of those social workers based in hospital settings continues to give cause for concern. This is not simply the result of the
changes of the NHS and Community Care Act 1990, it is a part of a
continuous debate about the location of one professional in the context of
another agency. Research undertaken in Scotland (Connor and Tibbitt,
1988) described the social work contribution as critical to collecting information (such as details of home circumstances), offering emotional support and co-ordinating discharge from hospital to support that was
acceptable and negotiated. In their view older people in geriatric wards
were likely to 'slip through the net' without social work intervention,
being particularly at risk if they lived on their own, while others were in
danger of drifting into residential care and a number proved to be under
pressure from their own caring responsibilities. Research on the impact
of the new proceedings under the NHS and Community Care Act 1990
(Rachman, 1995) suggests that hospital-based social workers are still
under increasing pressure to assess older patients. However, the focus of
this pressure has shifted so that assessment is concentrated on those who
appear likely to require intensive support, such as places in a nursing
home, residential care or regular domiciliary support. People who
appear to be managing or whose family appear to be supportive may be
more likely to rely on other services to discover hidden needs.

In essence the social work task revolves around assessment and care
management in settings such as hospitals and in provider arms of social
services departments. The British experience of care management has
been highly influenced by research into care management that focused on
older people at risk going into residential care in various locations
(Challis et al., 1988). The essence of the care management approach was to:
'enable social workers to develop sensitive and appropriate alternatives
to residential and long-term hospital care for frail elderly people' (Challis
et al., 1988, p. 14). These pilot projects argued that this mode of delivery of
community care provided significant benefits to the older people themselves, enhancing their choice and control, in line with their expressed
wishes to stay at home. The early projects gave front-line social workers
both smaller caseloads and control over a devolved budget to achieve
these aims (Challis and Davies, 1986).

In the 1980s case management and its successor, care management,
attracted official approval in both the Griffiths Report (1988) and the
White Paper, *Caring for People* (Department of Health, 1989). The latter

(p. 21) drew heavily on the Kent models in defining effective care management as:

- identification of people in need;
- assessment of care needs;
- planning and securing the delivery of care;
- monitoring the quality of care;
- reviewing clients' needs.

All the elements are visible in social services departments' implementation of the NHS and Community Care Act, although there are local variations of the organizational structure. One fundamental difference from the Kent model, however, exists in the extent to which social workers or care managers control budgets. (For a discussion of the variety of approaches see Orme and Glastonbury, 1993.) In practice, social workers in some areas are responsible for resource allocation mechanisms. As MacDonald and Myers (1995) have pointed out, this system appears to be much more responsive to service users' needs.

SOCIAL WORK AND ASSESSMENT

As described above, assessment is but one part of the care management process and is clearly not the totality of the social worker's role. However, in relation to working with older people in rehabilitation settings it is a key activity and it is useful to outline some of the general methods used in social work. This may be helpful for other professionals, whose own roles include responsibilities for individual assessments (see Chapter 7).

As a counterweight to the responsibilities and resources passed to local authorities under the NHS and Community Care Act 1990, the government has issued a range of detailed practitioner guidance. For example, the Social Services Inspectorate/Scottish Office (1991) have noted that assessment is a process of understanding 'an individual's needs and to relate them to agency policy and priorities, and to agree the objectives for any intervention' (p. 47). It is therefore more than a routinized collection of information and can vary in scope and duration.

Each local authority has developed its own local interpretation of such guidance and all have produced documentation to assist those undertaking assessments. All have also devised criteria for the various levels of assessment, e.g. for a bus pass, to complex or comprehensive assessment, e.g. for residential or nursing home care or intensive home-based services. To assist social workers in deciding the level of assessment needed by an individual, several stages may be involved, from referral to liaison with other professionals, to grading needs on a matrix (perhaps held on a computer).

Challis (1994) has pointed to the risk of overformularization and insensitivity (p. 71) in models of care management that neglect the relationships between professional and service user or service applicant.

For many social workers working with older people, there is a need to explore issues of loss and disability. Counselling skills can be used to develop relationships and increase the older person's sense of control and choice. Older people with dementia might be well served by social workers who are able to negotiate delicate balances between protection and risk taking.

Many of the principles of good assessment predate the NHS and Community Care Act 1990 and reflect social work values such as empowerment, anti-oppressive practice and normalization. Moreover, in relation to assessment of people who had applied to enter old people's homes, the National Institute for Social Work Unit (Neill, 1989) pointed to the dilemmas inherent in assessment when dealing with conflicts of interests and views between older people, their relatives and other professionals. Neill argued that assessment needs to bring forth the strengths and potential of older people, rather than being problem-focused. It also needs to be clear and honest about the extent of confidentiality.

Assessments by social workers are important both in determining need and in indicating possible responses to deficiencies of support. Each social services or social work department will have its own procedures and it is useful for other professionals to understand the content and process of assessment. Some authorities, for example, distinguish certain types of health problems for specialist assessment (i.e. assessments done by professionals experienced, say, in dementia or learning disabilities). Other distinguish assessments for those people in hospital by using hospital-based workers instead of community-based personnel. For those older people whose needs are being assessed this can doubtless be fairly confusing, but good practice in social work dictates that efforts are made to outline the procedure, to gain informed consent (e.g. about seeking information from third parties such as the GP or ward staff) and to let people know of their rights to complain.

The content of assessment may appear familiar to rehabilitation staff, focusing as it does on social circumstances, self-care abilities and disabilities, issues of risk and practical support. However, social workers also work in the context of financial charging for social care and so, unlike most other professionals in this area, they are required to assess individuals' financial circumstances and to explain that services may incur a charge. Whilst financial assessment has always been part of assessment for local authority residential care, it has been less prominent in day care and domiciliary services. Equally, as more older people now have savings, occupational pensions and disability benefits, they are facing charges for services. One key part of assessment lies in maintaining a relationship that can explore broad aspects of need and resources without being sucked into economically driven situations on either side. As Langan and Means (1995) have pointed out, the new culture of community care raises fundamental questions about people's rights to their own resources. Many social workers, while implementing charging policies, find this area difficult (Bradley and Manthorpe, 1995), particularly when they see individuals divesting themselves of assets to minimize charges but leaving themselves vulnerable to financial abuse. Alternatively, refusing to pay assessed charges may lead to non-receipt of services which may impinge on the rehabilitation efforts of other members of the team. Such decisions by the older person should be made on the basis of full information (see also Chapter 4).

As Taylor and Devine (1993, p. 10) have noted, assessment is the initial part of a helping cycle that can be broken into two parts: the gathering of information and the analysis of this information. There is currently a deal of emphasis on the policy context and procedural mechanisms associated with the implementation of the NHS and Community Care Act 1990. For social workers this may obscure other important skills, such as interview techniques, the handling of conflict and negotiation skills. Nonetheless, much social work practice continues to rely on these abilities to relate effectively to those undergoing assessment and carers or family members who are interested parties to the process. As Twigg and Atkin (1994) have related, the position of carers is often ambiguous in dealings with professionals. This is particularly so in social work practice where the distinctions between service users are frequently blurred. In assessing an individual who expresses a wish for a break from home, for example, the social worker will be mindful of the effect on the carer(s) involved and will have to assess the impact of such intervention on a range of matters from family dynamics to the family budget.

A completed assessment by a social worker may result in a number of outcomes. For older people whose needs are not assessed as significant or rather whose needs do not lie within the areas of priority of their particular social services authority, there may be no further action, although there might be helpful advice or referral to the health service, or voluntary or commercial sectors. For those individuals whose needs are given priority, the process of care management moves on to determining how best to meet those needs in the light of available resources and individual preferences.

SOCIAL WORK AND CARE CO-ORDINATION

This broad heading covers the delivery of social care services, co-ordinated by a care manager (who in this example is a social worker by profession). The key elements involve translating the findings of the assessment into planned and effective service delivery, which is monitored and revised to meet changing circumstances. As mentioned earlier the government's enthusiasm for care management was greatly influenced by the Kent experiments and this research emphasized the effectiveness of systems that gave care managers a degree of delegated responsibility. Their 'purse-holding' powers have not been commonly followed in other areas; in other words most social workers do not have a 'cheque book'.

Care managers nonetheless have responsibility to establish and support systems of service delivery in line with individual preferences and the budget allocated. For some individual older people who wish to move into residential or nursing home care this assistance may extend to maximizing choice, arranging visits or trial periods of residence, collecting information and arranging the move. Those who take a view that counselling is an integral part of their work may well focus on individual feelings of possible loss associated with the giving up of home, or possible anxiety about increasing dependency, or may get involved in helping people resolve troubling conflicts or past events. Such helping relationships may extend to other people, such as carers or family members. However, as Scrutton (1989) has pointed out, the counselling relationship is different from advice giving and the provision of services. It may well be that individual care managers take the view that while they can be supportive and inform their work with understanding of counselling principles they resist being seen as therapeutic workers. As much of this chapter has emphasized, the social work role is extremely elastic and is still open to discretion by the individuals concerned, in the context of the professional culture of their team and the organizational culture of their employing authority.

Care co-ordination has the potential for making major improvements in the lives of some older people. It is a system that stresses that services should be related to need and personal preferences, that services should be flexible and innovative and that the older person remains central in the web of provision with responsive services that are not wastefully duplicated. Other professionals will recognize the failings of previous systems whereby, for example, it was typically very difficult to arrange home care at weekends, or to decide agency responsibility for help with bathing or to identify the person responsible for having an overview of the older person's needs. The new system of care management attempts to deal with such frustrations, but it is important to note that there are still resource constraints on local authorities and, in many areas, new patterns of service have not developed.

Means and Smith (1994) commented that the community care reforms will be judged successful if they are perceived as appropriate and of high quality by users and carers (p. 134). Policy makers will also need to be convinced that they are efficient and publicly acceptable. While this book focuses on older people it is important to take account of the wider context of community care, particularly for younger people with mental health problems. Social and health care staff may be required to give this group priority, in order to respond to political and public disquiet. Such priority may move to one side the previous focus on older people, to the frustration of the multidisciplinary team.

SOCIAL WORK PROVISION

The sections above have concentrated on the social workers' role in the 'purchase' of social care for older people. We now move to discuss the skills employed by those social workers who provide services directly. In terms of location this type of work is to be found in day centres, residential and respite provision, work with individual older people and carers at home. Such work may be carried out by social services authorities, but is increasingly located in the voluntary, the not-for-profit and commercial sectors, since local authorities have been obliged to spend 85% of the money transferred to them on the full implementation of the NHS Community Care Act 1990 within the independent sector. As mentioned earlier some social workers are also 'attached' to health service facilities such as day hospitals, health centres, respite units or hospitals.

It may be useful to focus on some of the skills used by social workers in one particular activity, in order to draw out aspects of their professional work which may compare with others' practice. In this section the chosen activity is day services for older people with dementia, since this represents a service that is provided by many agencies and is probably familiar in many areas.

DAY SERVICES FOR PEOPLE WITH DEMENTIA

Twigg and Atkin (1994), in exploring policy and practice for the carers, noted that day care may be provided for people with dementia, but that its purpose is often related to the perceived needs of people's carers for support and respite. Thus the social work role within day care is not solely focused on the person who has a 'place' but can potentially include the carer and wider networks.

In a handbook written for residential and day care providers, Chapman, Jacques and Marshall (1994) drew out day-to-day issues that inevitably occur in providing individual care and care for a group in an artificial setting. The underlying values influencing the approaches adopted are likely to be familiar to many human service personnel, but social work training places particular emphasis on what it terms 'anti-oppressive practice'. Whilst this is often related to issues of race and gender, it has equal potential in work with older people and people with dementia, who may be disadvantaged and discriminated against on a variety of levels. Such an approach may help social workers in the debates about conflicts of interests, risk taking, the restriction of activity, sexuality and spiritual needs, all of which are covered by Chapman, Jacques and Marshall (1994) in more detail.

In terms of specific intervention, other social work skills may be usefully transferred to a day care setting. These can range from assistance with personal finances and welfare rights, which as Langan and Means (1995) demonstrated is a complicated area, to intensive therapeutic support for carers. At group level many social workers have also been involved in developing work in the area of reminiscence, alongside work on reality orientation, increasing social activities and opportunities for participation in wider community settings. Gibson (1994) illustrated the potential for highly specific reminiscence work with people who have dementia (see Chapter 8).

Social work in such settings is therefore not a discrete set of tasks but, as this brief description illustrates, the professional qualification has the **potential** to provide a sound synthesis of knowledge, skills and values for those service users who present particular challenges or face personal distress or dysfunction. The requirements for the Diploma in Social Work (CCETSW, 1991, p. 16) emphasize that professionals must be able to understand social and psychosocial processes and, more importantly perhaps, to seek to counteract the impact of 'stigma and discrimination'. They are specifically encouraged to address ageism in both policy and practice (CCETSW, 1992). Social work in day services with people who have dementia is clearly a fundamental test when such theories are put into practice.

CONCLUSION

It is probably infuriating for other professions to hear that an influential textbook for social work students claims that the stricture 'Social work is what social workers do' contains an element of truth, or more particularly that social work is what other professionals do not do (Hanvey and Philpot, 1994, p. 1). For many professionals working with other people this compartmentalism is being challenged by more holistic practice, although the vexed questions of accountability remain (Dalrymple and Burke, 1995). As we have seen, social workers work in a different organizational context from the majority of healthcare workers, with different legal imperatives. In rehabilitation work with older adults all professionals need a working knowledge of each others' potential contribution. At local level, all have a responsibility to build up systems of communication and effective patterns of practice. Concepts such as multidisciplinary assessments and inter-agency working have blurred the boundaries of professional knowledge and service delivery. Social work's strength lies not in its exclusive skill and knowledge base, but in its attention to the values and attitudes that permeate professional work with service users.

REFERENCES

Ahmad-Aziz, A., Froggatt, A., Richardson, I. *et al.* (1992) *Improving Practice with Elders*, Central Council for Education and Training in Social Work, London.

Biggs, S. (1993) *Understanding Ageing*, Open University Press, Buckingham.

Borsay, A. (1989) First child care, second mental health, third the elderly: professional education and the development of social work priorities. *Research Policy and Practice*, **7**(2), 22–30.

Bradley, G. and Manthorpe, J. (1995) The dilemmas of financial assessment: professional and ethical difficulties. *Practice*, **7**(4), 21–30.

CCETSW (1991) *Rules and Requirements for the Diploma in Social Work*, Central Council for Education and Training in Social Work, London.

CCETSW (1992) *Quality Work with Older People: Improving Social Work Education and Training*, Central Council for Education and Training in Social Work, London.

Challis, D. (1994) *Case management in Implementing Community Care* (ed N. Malin), Open University Press, Buckingham.

Challis, D. and Davies, B. (1986) *Case Management in Community Care*, Gower, Aldershot.

Challis, D., Chessum, R., Chesterman, J. *et al.* (1988) Community care for the frail elderly: an urban experiment. *British Journal of Social Work*, **18**(Supplement), 13–42.

Chapman, A., Jacques, A. and Marshall, M. (1994) *Dementia Care: A Handbook for Residential and Day Care*, Age Concern England, London.

Cheetham, J. (1993) Social work and community care in the 1990's, in *Social Policy Review* (eds R. Page and J. Baldock), Social Policy Association, Canterbury.

Clarke, J. (1993) The comfort of strangers: social work in context, in *A Crisis in Care? Challenges to Social Work* (ed J. Clarke), Sage, London.

Connor, A. and Tibbitt, J. (1988) *Social Workers and Health Care in Hospitals*, Scottish Office, HMSO, London.

Dalley, G. (1989) Professional ideology or organisational tribalism? The Health Service–social work divide, in *Social Work and Health Care* (eds R. Taylor and J. Ford), Jessica Kingsley Publishers, London.

Dalley, G. (1991) Beliefs and behaviour: professionals and the policy process. *Journal of Aging Studies*, **5**(2), 163–80.

Dalrymple, J. and Burke, B. (1995) *Anti-Oppressive Practice; Social Care and the Law*, Open University Press, Buckingham.

Davis Smith, J., Rochester, C. and Hedley, R. (eds) (1995) *An Introduction to the Voluntary Sector*, Routledge, London.

Department of Health (1989) *Caring for People: Community Care in the Next Decade and Beyond*, Cm 849, HMSO, London.

Gibson, F. (1994) What can reminiscence contribute to people with dementia? in *Reminiscence Reviewed* (ed J. Bornat), Open University Press, Buckingham.

Griffiths, R. (1988) *Community Care: An Agenda for Action*, HMSO, London.

Grimwood, C. and Popplestone, R. (1993) *Women, Management and Care*, Macmillan, London.

Hanvey, C. and Philpot, T. (eds) (1994) *Practising Social Work*, Routledge, London.

Hugman, R. (1991) *Power in Caring Professions*, Macmillan, London.

Hunter, D. (1988) Meeting the challenge of coordinated service delivery, in *Mental Health Problems in Old Age* (eds B. Gearing, M. Johnson and T. Heller), John Wiley and Sons, Chichester.

Hutchinson, A. and Gordon, S. (1992) Primary care teamwork – making it a reality. *Journal of Interprofessional Care*, 6(1), 31–42.

Langan, J. and Means, R. (1995) *Personal Finances, Elderly People with Dementia and the 'New' Community Care*. Anchor Housing Association, Kidlington.

Langan, M. and Day, L. (eds) (1992) *Women, Oppression and Social Work*, Routledge, London.

Lee-Treewick, G. (1994) Bedroom abuse: the hidden work in a nursing home. *Generations Review*, 4(2), 2–4.

Lewis, J. (1993) Community care: policy imperatives, joint planning and enabling authorities. *Journal of Interprofessional Care*, 7(1), 7–14.

MacDonald, C. and Myers, F. (1995) *Assessment and Care Management: The Practitioner Speaks*. University of Stirling Social Work Research Centre, Stirling.

Manthorpe, J,. and Hettiaratchy, P. (1993) Multi-disciplinary learning – a pilot project. *Journal of Educational Gerontology*, 8(2), 86–99.

Manthorpe, J. and Stanley, N. (1996) Private placements; opportunity or oppression. *Social Work Education*, 15(4), in press.

Marshall, M. (1989) *Working with Dementia*, Venture Press, Birmingham.

Means, R. and Smith, R. (1994) *Community Care: Policy and Practice*, Macmillan, London.

Neill, J. (1989) *Assessing Elderly People for Residential Care: A Practical Guide*, National Institute for Social Work Research Unit, London.

Nocon, A. (1994) *Collaboration in Community Care in the 1990's*, Business Education Publishers, Sunderland.

Orme, J. and Glastonbury, B. (1993) *Care Management*, Macmillan, London.

Phillips, J. (1992) *Private Residential Care: The Admission Process and Reactions of the Public Sector*, Avebury, Aldershot.

Phillipson, C. and Biggs, S. (1992) *Understanding Elder Abuse: A Training Manual for Helping Professionals*, Longman, Harlow.

Pietroni, P. (1992) Towards reflective practice – the language of health and social care. *Journal of Interprofessional Care*, 6(1), 7–16.

Pritchard, S. and Brearley, P. (1982) Risk and social work, in *Risk and Ageing* (ed C.P. Brearley), Routledge and Kegan Paul, London.

Rachman, R. (1995) Community care: changing the role of hospital social work. *Journal of Health and Social Care in the Community*, 3(2), 163–72.

Scrutton, S. (1989) *Counselling Older People*, Edward Arnold, London.

Social Services Inspectorate/Scottish Office (1991) *Care Management and Assessment: Practitioners' Guide*, HMSO, London.

Taylor, B. and Devine, T. (1993) *Assessing Needs and Planning Care in Social Work*, Arena, Aldershot.

Tinker, A. (1992) *Elderly People in Modern Society*, 3rd edn, Longman, Harlow.

Twigg, J. and Atkin, K. (1994) *Carers Perceived*, Open University Press, Buckingham.

Walker, A. (1993) Poverty and inequality in old age, in *Ageing in Society* (eds J. Bond, P. Coleman and S. Peace), Sage, London.

Wright, F., Ball, C. and Coleman, P. (1988) *Collaboration in Care*, Age Concern England, Surrey.

Yelloly, M. (1995) Professional competence and higher education, in *Learning and Teaching in Social Work: Towards Reflective Practice* (eds M. Yelloly and M. Henkel), Jessica Kingsley Publishers, London.

Physiotherapy with older people

13

Jane Stephenson

INTRODUCTION

Physiotherapists are health professionals who emphasize the use of physical approaches in the prevention and treatment of disease and disability. They deal with problems associated with the musculoskeletal, neuromuscular, cardiovascular and respiratory systems.

The Chartered Society of Physiotherapy is the recognized professional body for physiotherapists in the United Kingdom and is responsible for the setting and maintenance of standards (CSP, 1990); it is an autonomous body, setting its own rules of professional conduct. Chartered physiotherapists undertake a recognized course of work leading to a degree-level qualification.

The curriculum undertaken by chartered physiotherapists covers human anatomy and physiology, diseases and disabilities, assessment of movement and function, goal setting and treatment planning, evaluation of treatment, research methodology and treatment methods such as massage, manipulation and movement techniques and the use of electrotherapy modalities. In acquiring these skills physiotherapists are ideally placed to identify and help solve movement problems and also to help prevent problems and act as educators in the health promotion role.

Once qualified, physiotherapists usually gain experience working in the National Health Service. Over a period of up to two years they work in many different areas, for example out-patients, paediatrics, elderly care, surgery, orthopaedics and community. After this period they generally look to gain more responsible posts, often concentrating on developing their expertise in a particular field. Physiotherapists can be found working with all age groups in many different places, for example hospitals (NHS and private), schools, general practitioners' surgeries, people's own homes, physiotherapy private practice, residential and nursing homes (CSP, 1992) and industry.

A prerequisite for physiotherapists working in the NHS is that they must be state registered physiotherapists (SRP). State registration takes place on an annual basis and the register of names is kept by the Council for Professions Supplementary to Medicine. Registration can be withdrawn for breaches of professional conduct. As independent practitioners physiotherapists take full responsibility for their own professional practice.

OLDER PEOPLE

The standard definition of 'old age' in the United Kingdom is pensionable age, which is currently 60 years for women and 65 years for men. We are living in an increasingly ageing population, but many people who are aged 60 and over or indeed 80 and over do not think of themselves as old and lead active lives, rarely having to be involved with any health professionals. Old age is often assumed to be linked with frailty, disability and cognitive impairment which is not necessarily the case. Age can also engender negative attitudes to rehabilitation potential. Nieuwboer (1992) found that 'stereotypes might have a profound effect on the quality of older patients' treatment' and influence the provision of physiotherapy even though the 'fundamental principles on which physiotherapy practice is based apply equally to people of all ages including older people' (ACPSIEP, 1991).

Physiotherapists working specifically with older people develop their skills to help take the older person through their particular problem and achieve their optimum function and independence, whilst recognizing that the ageing process can reduce the efficiency of the body's systems.

Older people can be divided into several groups in terms of their contact with physiotherapists:

1. Those older people who never see a physiotherapist, because they either do not perceive the need or do not actually have a need;
2. Older people who have a one-off problem and see a physiotherapist with particular expertise in that area, for example someone with back pain visiting a physiotherapist as an out-patient. The problem is dealt with as a completed episode;
3. Older people who are experiencing a greater assault to the body, for example a stroke, an amputation, or major surgery. These people will be seen in the hospital or home setting, although not necessarily in a designated 'older care' setting;
4. Older people who are experiencing multiple pathology as well as the natural ageing process; for example, a person with an existing amputation may subsequently have a stroke; the stroke patient may already be severely disabled by osteoarthritis. These people are often

the ones seen in the designated older care facility, such as the elderly care unit in a hospital or the day hospital, where the relevant expertise exists;
5. The very frail older person with multiple pathology needing help from carers to maintain their function whether at home, in a residential home or nursing home.

The true expertise of the physiotherapist working with older people lies in the last two groups, where there is the presentation of multiple pathology with the ageing process. The physiotherapist working with the older person is skilled in assessing the problems present, and in defining any new movement problem in a body that may already have physical limitations or mental health problems (Pomeroy, 1994). The nature of this multiple problem presentation makes it very difficult to be prescriptive about the treatment programme. The physiotherapist will then provide the necessary intervention, whether it be in the form of direct treatment, or teaching a carer or other members of the multi-disciplinary team. It is also a skill to recognize when physiotherapy intervention is not going to be of help. Physiotherapists who combine their knowledge of the function of the human body with an under-standing of and empathy with the ageing process are well placed to solve the mobility problems of the older person and gain their maximum independence; to maintain that position or, when this is no longer possible, to assist in keeping the older person as comfortable and pain free as possible.

Physiotherapists are also ideally suited to teach the carers of older people, whether they be members of the family or the multidisciplinary team, how best to assist the person with multiple disability, or perhaps **not** to assist but to allow the older person to use their own skills in their own time.

REFERRAL

Older people can refer themselves for physiotherapy; however, in most areas there will be a recognized referral system and criteria for referral. In all cases the physiotherapist will liaise with relevant members of the healthcare team. In many hospital settings a 'blanket referral scheme' exists where the physiotherapist undertakes to see each patient admitted to the ward or unit and following assessment provides a treatment plan including intervention if necessary. It should be recognized that a referral is not prescriptive of treatment; the physiotherapist will make an assess-ment and only then can a decision be made as to whether physiotherapy intervention is suitable or not. A standard time between receiving the referral and carrying out the assessment should be indicated.

THE TEAM

Physiotherapists in most situations work as part of a team (see also Chapter 6). They may be members of a larger physiotherapy department within a hospital or, if in private practice working single-handed, they may be in contact with other private practitioners and colleagues in other disciplines. Clinical interest groups exist within the Chartered Society of Physiotherapy and bring together physiotherapists working in the same field; for example, for physiotherapists working specifically with older people there is the Association of Chartered Physiotherapists with a Special Interest in Elderly People (ACPSIEP, now called AGILE). These groups facilitate support for their members both regionally and nationally, through courses and conferences. They also publish journals and national standards of practice, and promote research.

Physiotherapists will also be members of the multidisciplinary team in primary (Gibson, 1988) and secondary care. They should be aware of the other members of the team and the skills that they bring to bear on the patient. They should also be aware of the role of the other team members and liaise with them whenever necessary.

Team working is an important aspect of the care of the older person, especially those who are experiencing multiple problems as described earlier. Many people can be involved in the treatment of the patient whether in their own home or in the hospital setting and optimum results can only be achieved if the team have agreed their intervention and goals.

Whenever the older person comes into contact with the physiotherapist the following process should occur:

- examination and assessment
- goal setting
- treatment plan
- review.

EXAMINATION AND ASSESSMENT

BACKGROUND INFORMATION

It is essential that certain information is obtained to build up a picture of the older person prior to the physiotherapy examination and assessment. This background information will include obvious details – name, address, date of birth, general practitioner, consultant, also relevant medical and social history and medication. The patient should not be expected to repeat information that has already been given to another member of the team and is easily accessible by the physiotherapist. The details gained can have a bearing on physiotherapy intervention, goal setting and outcome. The patient's medical history may have a bearing on their present problem or contraindicate some forms of physiotherapy intervention.

A record of the patient's social history is essential. For instance, do they live in a house where they have to cope with stairs and a bathroom upstairs? Does the older person have anyone at home who can help them or do they need to be informed of agencies they can apply to for help? Do they already receive help from any agencies, in which case does this need changing, or do the helpers need to be contacted to inform them of, say, a specific handling method?

The physiotherapist should be aware of the medication that the patient is taking and have a general understanding of the effects of certain groups of medicines and how they may affect treatment and physical function.

After as much information as possible has been gathered, the examination and assessment specific to physiotherapy can be undertaken.

PHYSIOTHERAPY

A subjective history is taken to identify the problems as seen by the older person. This should identify their previous level of ability and their expectations of recovery. During this time it should be possible to make an evaluation of the older person's personal care, communication abilities, posture, expressions, mood and motivation, all of which can have a bearing on the actual physical examination, possible intervention and outcome (Hastings, 1994).

This is followed by an objective examination where the physiotherapist uses knowledge of structure and function of the human body to identify any physical cause for the presenting symptoms (see also Chapter 6). The process of examination and assessment often highlights other areas that are not perceived by the older person to be a problem, but could be the underlying cause of their symptoms; for example, a painful knee can have its origins in the hip joint or lumbar spine. Where specific problems are found, standard measurements should be made for joint range, balance reactions, pain level, and so on.

Assessment may take place over several sessions according to the patient's state of health, level of communication, tolerance of the examination, intervention by other team members, and so on. However, at the end of each session and at the end of the full examination and assessment the results should be discussed if possible with the patient. Short- and long-term goals are then set with the older person and/or their carers and explanation given on the intervention necessary to achieve these goals.

COMMUNICATION

During the examination and assessment procedure the physiotherapist will make a judgement on the language and communication skills of the patient, as this will have an important bearing on the intervention used (see also Chapter 9). The older person may have their language and communication affected by a stroke and this can result in them not being able to express themselves clearly or accurately or not being able to understand what is being said by the physiotherapist. This can affect the information gathered by the physiotherapist and can also affect their explanation of the intervention to be used and the goals to be attained. Physiotherapy involves much 'hands on' treatment and can require close contact with the person involved, often moving into their personal space. If this happens without an adequate attempt to establish some form of contact, the intervention could be frightening, or cause stress and anxiety. In some cases where adequate communication is not possible but physiotherapy intervention is considered essential, explanation is still important and should be given to the patient and also their carer/advocate. In all cases it is extremely important that the rights of the older person are protected and that their personal autonomy is maintained as far as possible (see also Chapter 4).

GOAL SETTING

Goals set can be short and long term, for example, short term to reduce pain from acute injury, long term to restore optimum function of the affected area. Goals set should be realistic for the patient to achieve but at the same time set a challenge. Skill is needed in agreeing the optimum. Physiotherapists are often over-ambitious in their expectations (see also Chapter 4). Some patients are unrealistic in their expectations or unwilling or unable to come to terms with some aspects of their disability (see also Chapters 4 and 8). Where on examination the physiotherapist has perceived other problems that the patient has not discussed, these need to be highlighted to see if the patient wishes to address these as well. Where necessary the carer of the older person should be involved in the goal setting process. At all times, the decision of the patient and/or their carer should be based on full information about the intervention and their contribution, and the consequences of non-consent.

INTERVENTION

Physiotherapists will apply appropriate techniques to the physical problem presented. There are many techniques and not just one will apply to a particular situation. It is important that the physiotherapist reviews the treatment regularly and rechecks the objective markers high-lighted in the examination and assessment. It may be that if one treatment modality is not giving the required result after a complete episode, a further modality should be tried. It is also important that the physio-therapist is able to recognize any areas where their skills may be limited and to liaise with other therapists who are skilled in this area, in order to provide the optimum treatment for the patient. Physiotherapists are continually striving to improve their treatment techniques and to add new ones to their repertoire – they have recently been referred to as 'The Orthodox Alternative' as many physiotherapists are undertaking to learn some of the complementary therapies as part of their post-registration training (CSP, undated). This means that some chartered physiotherapists are competent to offer treatments such as acupuncture, aromatherapy and reflextherapy to their patients.

HOME ASSESSMENT

During the period of physiotherapy intervention, whether the patient is an in-patient, day hospital patient, or is seen at another venue away from the home, an assessment of the home situation could be required. This should be undertaken by members of the team relevant to the situation with appropriate joint discussion beforehand and afterwards. The purpose of the assessment will be appropriate to the pattern of life that the patient will wish to return to, and the availability of support systems. The long- and short-term goals, together with the treatment plan, will be formulated in response to these observations and in discussion with patient, carer and colleagues.

AUDIT

Physiotherapists will be involved in auditing their input with the patient, whether it be looking at an intradisciplinary function such as the objective measures they are using for their physiotherapy intervention, or multi-disciplinary such as the process of discharge from a hospital ward. Zinober (1995) describes audit as 'a systematic method of delivering high quality care through objectively reviewing practice, setting targets and managing and monitoring their implementation'.

WALKING AIDS

A result of the assessment undertaken by the physiotherapist could be the prescription of a walking aid. Walking aids may be a short-term issue to help someone mobilize whilst gaining muscle power in their leg or to help them balance whilst they are in plaster of Paris. They may be a long-term issue, for example for the patient with rheumatoid arthritis or the stroke patient with a permanent deficit.

Walking aids take many forms, shapes and sizes – sticks, walking frames, rollator frames, elbow crutches, axillary crutches. They should be adjusted to the correct size before issue and checked that they are safe. It is important that they are not seen as the complete solution to a problem and it is also important that they are issued by someone, such as a physiotherapist, with good knowledge of their effects, benefits and problems. A walking aid issued incorrectly can not only be of danger to the person using it but can also be detrimental to their recovery from a movement problem. Many visits to the homes of older people will result in the discovery of a wide selection of walking aids, some discarded because they were not of use, some inappropriately 'handed on' to others, and some adapted to meet other needs such as a clothes airer! A survey undertaken by Simpson and Pirrie (1991) found that out of 124 walking aids used by elderly people less than one-third were suitable and that chartered physiotherapists were the most successful suppliers of correct walking aids.

It is essential that the physiotherapist issuing a walking aid checks not only that it is of the correct height and can be used safely but also that the environment in which the walking aid is to be used is appropriate. Many walking frames, for instance, are ideal when used on the hospital ward but a hazard when taken home and placed in a room where there are loose carpets or an excess of furniture. If the problem is not fully assessed the walking aid will act only as a temporary prop whilst the underlying condition probably deteriorates. For example, an older person could be experiencing falls due to a weakness around the knee joint and they need to be given exercises to do as well as being provided with the walking aid to help them through the period of lessened mobility.

The physiotherapist must keep up to date in their knowledge of the walking aids available on the market. Some aids can be issued through hospital loan schemes; others have to be bought by the patient. The physiotherapist should be aware of what is available on the loan scheme and if they think that aids being issued are out of date or have been discarded due to a safety feature they should endeavour to notify the manager for an improvement. This is often a failing in a large health service organization, where it becomes 'habit' to keep the same item in stock. In terms of private purchase of walking aids, the chartered physiotherapist risks infringing the professional code of ethics by recommending one particular outlet or trade name, but should be aware of what is available and keep an up-to-date selection of brochures for the patient to look through, giving help as required. In many settings this can be done in conjunction with colleagues working in occupational therapy within both health and social services (see also Chapter 14). Many areas of the country now have Disabled Living Centres, where a wide range of aids are kept and can be tried out to test suitability before purchase is made.

The prescription and issue of aids must be clearly documented and it must be made clear that it is the responsibility of the user to check for safety issues once the aid is in their care. Many hospital departments ask for documents to be signed by the user of the aid, indicating that they have been instructed in the correct and safe use of the aid and are taking responsibility for checking certain safety issues that will have been pointed out by the person issuing the aid.

WHEELCHAIRS

As with walking aids, wheelchairs are pieces of equipment that should not be issued as the complete solution to the problem; they form part of the problem solving package. According to place of work, availability of staff and 'historical background' wheelchairs are issued by several members of the multidisciplinary team, physiotherapists and occupational therapists being the main professions associated with this work (see also Chapter 14). Physiotherapists should have knowledge of wheelchairs available both via the health service and privately. They should be aware of the assessment procedure in choosing the most suitable chair and where they are not fully competent in these skills they should seek advice. In most areas the wheelchair allocation process has been centralized to a specialist Wheelchair Centre where referrals can be made.

Physiotherapists can then be involved in teaching the patient and/or carer how to use the chair. This involves knowing about the wheelchair mechanisms and how they work, the optimum way to manoeuvre the chair, how to dismantle and store the chair, and how to lift it correctly without causing back problems.

ORTHOSES

Orthoses are used as aids to assist in gaining optimum position and movement. Under this heading comes the issue of splints, shoes, insoles for shoes, and so on. It will depend on the location and staffing as to who takes this role. It could be that one person is responsible or it could be that the role is shared with different professions taking the lead according to the problem or location of the patient. In any of these cases the physiotherapist should still have a knowledge of the orthoses available and the effects that they have and they should liaise closely with the person issuing the orthosis. It cannot be too strongly emphasized that an orthosis is unlikely to be the total answer to the problem and it may be a long- or short-term need. For example, a splint may be used to give support whilst treatment is taking place to increase muscle power or reduce pain and when the goal is reached the splint can be discarded. Alternatively, someone with a foot problem following a stroke may not gain full return of function and need a suitable orthosis to hold the foot in the correct position to give them the optimum safe gait pattern (see also Chapter 11).

THE FUTURE

Advances in technology and medical care mean that people are living to a greater age, many of them fit and active, others surviving illness and injury and having to cope with disability. Changes in healthcare are meaning a move from the 'stay in hospital'; we now have day surgery, earlier discharges to the home setting and treatment entirely in the home setting. People are expected to take more responsibility for their own health, either by health prevention measures or by carrying out their own treatment programmes unsupervised, with intermittent assessment and intervention by the healthcare professional. Greater demand is also being placed on the carers of older people to maintain frail disabled people in their own homes, or residential and nursing homes. In return for these expected responsibilities, older people and their carers are seeking a more influential role in the assessment, planning and service delivery process.

Physiotherapists are ideally placed to be key workers in this environment. They have the ability to assess and set up short and long term plans to deal with mobility problems in whatever environment these may occur. Physiotherapists are skilled teachers and can therefore take part in health promotion and in teaching carers of older people.

In order to fulfil their potential in this future picture, physiotherapists must continue to monitor their practice, using tools such as the quality cycle, clinical audit and research. They must make sure that their interventions are efficient, relevant and effective and that where appropriate they delegate tasks to others they have trained (Simpson, 1993).

The physiotherapy curriculum must keep up to date with the pace of change and its content be reviewed to include only relevant and proven techniques and the use of up-to-date technology in terms of equipment used both for intervention with the patient and for information technology.

At the time of writing this chapter the physiotherapy profession has been in existence for 100 years. The next 100 years will see physiotherapists challenged to use their already proven skills and recognize the need for change (Squires, 1995).

REFERENCES

ACPSIEP (1991) *Physiotherapy with Older People: Standards of Clinical Practice*, Chartered Society of Physiotherapy, London.

CSP (1990) *Standard of Physiotherapy Practice*, Chartered Society of Physiotherapy, London.

CSP (1992) *Physiotherapy with Older People in Long Stay Care*, Briefing Paper no. 13, Chartered Society of Physiotherapy, London.

CSP (undated) *Physiotherapy: The Orthodox Alternative*, Chartered Society of Physiotherapy, London.

Gibson, A. (ed) (1988) *Physiotherapy in the Community*, Woodhead Faulkner, Cambridge.

Hastings, M. (1994) *The Role of Physiotherapy in the Post Acute Care of Older People*, Presentation to the Royal College of Physicians, London.

Nieuwboer, A.M. (1992) Attitudes towards working with older patients: physiotherapists' responses to video presentations of post amputation gait training for an older and a younger patient. *Physiotherapy Theory and Practice*, 8(1), 27–37.

Pomeroy, V.M. (1994) Mobility, dementia and rehabilitation. *Physiotherapy and Practice*, 10(1), 35–43.

Simpson, J.M. (1993) Physiotherapy with older people: recommendations for further development. *Physiotherapy Theory and Practice*, 9(1), 53–5.

Simpson, C. and Pirrie, L. (1991) Walking aids: a survey of suitability and supply. *Physiotherapy*, 77(3), 231–4.

Squires, A. (1995) Future directions for the role of the physiotherapist in the care and treatment of older people, in *Physiotherapy with Older People* (eds B. Pickles *et al.*), Saunders, London.

Zinober, B.W. (1995) Reflections on the development of audit. *Physiotherapy*, 81(4), 175–6.

Occupational therapy with older people 14

Jean Hall

INTRODUCTION

There have been a number of significant developments in the role of the occupational therapist during the past 25 years (COT, 1990a). The Chronically Sick and Disabled Persons Act 1970 was the stimulus to move from mainly hospital work settings into local authority social service (community) departments. A major influence underpinning much of the subsequent legislation during this time has been perceived as the needs of an ageing population. The shortfall between supply and demand for occupational therapists has been documented in numerous reports (for example, Blom-Cooper, 1989).

Considerable attempts have been made during the past five years to redress the shortage of qualified occupational therapists. One example is that the degree-based training courses are becoming more adaptable to accommodate mature, part-time students. However, there is a continual need to encourage ongoing finance for additional training places, and to promote new initiatives and incentives which will entice back to work the therapists who have left (COT, 1994a).

Occupational therapy assistants/helpers have been part of the service for some time. They do not have a professional occupational therapy qualification and their work must be supervised by staff who do (COT, 1990b). They are encouraged to participate in in-service training and appropriate short courses, which enhance their skills and motivation. Helpers have different grades to reflect the level of responsibility they have been trained to undertake.

STANDARDS OF PRACTICE

The College of Occupational Therapists continues to publish and update standards, policies and procedures documents on a wide range of important professional issues (COT, 1995).

Key areas of work for the occupational therapist with older people are:

- hospital-based rehabilitation
- wheelchair services
- community/local authority-based resettlement.

THE HOSPITAL-BASED OCCUPATIONAL THERAPIST

In the hospital setting, the focus is on assessing patients who have become acutely ill, or who have been affected by traumatic accidents. Once a careful assessment has been carried out, a treatment plan is developed in conjunction with the patient, carer and other disciplines (Turner, 1992). This takes into account the patient's needs and wishes (SSI, 1991), as well as any contraindications that must be considered. The assessment should identify the patient's main strengths and problems, and if applicable a treatment programme should be prepared and modified as necessary during a continuing assessment. The programme will focus on personal, domestic and social aspects of the patient's life as well as psychological and physical factors (SSI, 1991).

Treatment includes carefully planned programmes of graded activities, selected to meet the specific needs of the patient and to lead to their rehabilitation and discharge (Turner, 1992). The programme is likely to include a selection of the following, some of which overlap with other disciplines. A lead professional may be selected to ensure continuity and avoid gaps and duplications.

General mobility indoors
- standing and sitting, checking the most suitable height and design of chair or stool;
- getting into bed, lying down, turning over, sitting up and getting out of bed;
- method of transferring from bed to chair or commode or wheelchair, and back again;
- mobility, whether walking unaided, with assistance, with a frame or in a wheelchair indoors;
- managing steps and stairs, noting the need for handrails or other assistance.

Personal hygiene
- washing upper part of body;
- washing lower part of body;
- brushing teeth with toothpaste; or
- washing dentures, as appropriate;

- shaving;
- cutting fingernails and toenails;
- using the toilet and managing clothing;
- adjusting incontinence pads or other aids to personal comfort and hygiene;
- using a shower; or
- using a bath, perhaps with a need for assistance and/or special equipment.

Household management and food preparation
- selection of household tasks, beginning with simple everyday ones and progressing to more complicated ones;
- preparation of simple snacks and drinks, with the patient encouraged to think about a balanced diet;
- preparation of cooked meals, ensuring that patient has adequate skills to continue cooking when discharged home; or
- discussion with the patient about acceptable alternatives; these may include frozen meals, a microwave oven, meals on wheels, assistance from a good neighbour or home carer.

It may also be appropriate to discuss with the patient other activities such as hobbies and cultural or leisure pursuits, and to assist in their achievement. For example, a patient who has been a keen gardener may no longer be able to carry out heavy tasks in the garden (Please, 1990), but may happily continue to grow plants from seed and use a greenhouse, garden shed or window ledge.

Activities such as horticulture and cookery provide very sociable small group activities within the department, providing the occupational therapist with opportunities to observe interaction, levels of concentration, sociability and levels of ability. Members of the group will often provide encouragement to a newcomer or someone who lacks confidence.

Essential skills of the occupational therapist include the ability to listen and observe carefully, being aware and sensitive to the older person (Burnard, 1989); to appreciate the effect on them of their altered circumstances and environment; to conceptualize whether the patient is likely to be able to manage independently at home, or what assistance may be required and from whom. Pressure for increasing patient throughput may result in rehabilitative treatment being continued in the community, with consequent costs to the service (see Chapter 1).

THE WHEELCHAIR SERVICE

Since April 1991, wheelchair provision under the NHS has been delegated to District Health Authorities to commission. Services provided at these units vary throughout the UK; ideally they should have a sufficient number of qualified physiotherapists and occupational therapists, medical, technical and other support staff to enable a comprehensive service to be provided. Although wheelchairs can be prescribed by general practitioners, a full assessment by trained professionals is recommended for cost-effective provision and training.

Professionals must have a comprehensive understanding of the total lifestyle and the physical, psychological and practical needs of the user for whom they are prescribing. The wheelchair should be understood as a means of mobility for those with limited or no walking ability. For those persons who of necessity spend a considerable part of their day in a wheelchair, it is essential that features other than mobility are catered for. Most importantly the needs of full seating support must be assessed, taking into account medical, physical, postural and management needs.

The therapist will need to understand the client's abilities and needs as perceived at the time of assessment, and to consider aspects of daily living which may be improved by selecting the most appropriate seating to suit the individual. The therapist must also take into account the abilities of the carer(s) when assisting the client in the home environment, when travelling or in other ways specific to that person.

To ensure that the needs of the individual are fully understood it will be necessary for the therapist to visit the user in the home environment, and to spend sufficient time assessing how they will manage or be managed in their own setting. The assessment may also consider how the wheelchair will be used outdoors and how the user will be able to be transported with their chair when necessary.

ASPECTS OF THE ASSESSMENT TO BE CONSIDERED

The primary aim of any referral is to ensure that the user may be provided with wheeled mobility which takes account of essential orthopaedic and therapeutic objectives of comfort and ability to function throughout the day; this should take account of the need to alter posture and to be appropriately supported in different positions.

For short journeys where the client is, for example, going or being pushed to the local shops, an upright sitting position with a basic cushion may be sufficient. A user with more complex needs may require a seating system that consists of trunk support and a forward tilting seat with a knee cushion. Where there are spinal or postural deformities, the seating specification must make allowance for these, otherwise the client will not only be uncomfortable but also at increased risk of pressure sores and further anatomical deterioration. It may be advisable to adjust the client's position at certain times of the day, to improve circulation and comfort by providing a chair with reclining and semi-reclining features.

THE PRESCRIPTION

When prescribing, the wheelchair therapist should consider the following.

- The reason for the referral and by whom it has been made;
- The wishes or perceptions of the patient/client. The occupational therapist must be sensitive to the client's feelings about using a wheelchair when faced with using one for the first time;
- The role played by the carer(s) and their wishes or perceptions.

The above three points may be influenced by how much knowledge/experience the client and carer have of wheelchairs.

- If the client is already using a wheelchair, the therapist should consider how this is being used and any aspects which should be altered or improved.
- The client's age, general health and strength should be noted, along with any contraindications, e.g. is the client physically fit to be using a self-propelled chair?

ENVIRONMENTAL CONSTRAINTS

The therapist should take a detailed description of likely physical and environmental constraints on the prescription. A home visit is probably the only certain method of ensuring that this is fully accurate, and the following points should be noted.

- The geographical location of the client's home;
- The topographical features of where they live;
- Parking space and restrictions;
- Parked vehicles and traffic adjacent to the dwelling;
- Access from the road to the environs of the home, noting any uneven surfaces, steps, slopes, shared pathways, gateways and paths to the front door, etc.;
- Accessibility of the client's home, noting doorway widths and steps (dimensions, construction and condition);

- Egress from the dwelling, in case of emergency or to enter the rear garden, looking at pathways and other features necessary to the client's use of those facilities;
- Space constraints within the home, in respect of turning space to enter and leave rooms, doorways, projecting radiators, furniture or other space constraints;
- Floor coverings/surfaces/loose mats or anything that will impede or endanger the client;
- Location of essential facilities, kitchen, bathroom/WC, telephone, etc.;
- Potential hazards.

It is also advisable for the occupational therapist to note the requirements of other people who live or visit the premises, including children and animals.

The therapist will need to spend time with the client/carer, going through the normal daily routine and identifying any special features that must be incorporated into the wheelchair prescription.

SOME QUESTIONS TO BE CONSIDERED FOR INDOOR USE

How long will the client spend in the wheelchair?
What other seating is available and how appropriate is it?
How will the client transfer to and from the wheelchair?
What kind of bed is used and how will the client transfer to and from it?
Where is the WC and bathroom and how will transfers be effected?
If a hoist is to be used, is it compatible with using the wheelchair?
Who will assist and have they been trained?
Is there a stairlift? If so, is it one that will carry a person in a wheelchair?
If a stairlift is to be installed, will there be adequate space and facilities for carrying a wheelchair safely? What help is available if the client gets into difficulties?
Is there a telephone or call-alarm system easily available?
What safety precautions are in evidence, e.g. in the kitchen?
What security systems have been installed?
What arrangements are in place for night-time care? This is particularly relevant where the client lives alone, and may be dependent on one or a number of carers, nurses, etc.
Daytime activities should be considered; for example does the client go out and by what means?
Are other forms of transport used and if so what are they?
Are there additional features, such as a safety harness, required within that other vehicle?

WHEELCHAIR PROVISION

There are many types of wheelchair from which to select (Male and Massie, 1990; DLF, current edition); they are not, however, all available from the District Wheelchair Service. Powered wheelchairs for outdoor use are seldom provided under the NHS scheme. The following options should be considered.

Self-propelled, attendant-propelled (Griffiths and Wynne, 1991), attendant-propelled with power assistance; powered indoor, powered outdoor wheelchairs.

Indoor use only, outdoor use only, dual use.

Dimensions when open, dimensions when folded, and weight.

Pneumatic or solid tyres.

Removable components, and whether the chair has to be dismantled for transportation in another vehicle.

Ease of use, and ease of stowing into boot of a car or by car-hoist.

Stability of chair in use and under extreme circumstances, such as being used on steps and kerbs.

Adjustability and positioning of footrests, armrests and backrest to accommodate seating requirements.

Availability of appropriate and compatible seating inserts, cushions, etc.

Availability of optional extras such as lap-straps, trays, or specially designed additions to suit specific individuals.

Once the prescribed chair and seating system is available, the occupational therapist must ensure that the client and/or carers are able to use it safely and that they understand how to deal with maintenance and repairs and, where appropriate, how to obtain comprehensive insurance cover.

THE SOCIAL SERVICE BASED OCCUPATIONAL THERAPIST

The role of the occupational therapist working in a social services department of a local authority is different from, but complementary to, that of their colleague working in an NHS trust. While the latter will be responsible for treatment and rehabilitation programmes and discharge plans, the social services occupational therapist will be responsible for resettlement if the patient is being discharged home, and for facilitating independent living or care with dignity for the disabled person.

The responsibilities in working for a local authority social services department will vary in scope between different local authorities in the UK. These differences will depend upon such things as:

> - the size of the local authority;
> - whether it is a borough or a county council;
> - the political colour of the local authority;
> - the commitment of the elected members on the social services committee, and of the officers, to meeting the needs of disabled persons and older persons, and to the employment of occupational therapists;
> - the availability and allocation of finance and resources;
> - the availability of suitably qualified occupational therapists, given the national shortfall of qualified staff.

The common link between occupational therapists, whether hospital or social services based, and colleagues in the other professions allied to medicine is their similar basic professional education.

THE ROLE OF THE LOCAL AUTHORITY OCCUPATIONAL THERAPIST

The role of the occupational therapist based in a social services department will complement that of colleagues working in health services. Immediate colleagues are likely to be other occupational therapists and assistants, possibly a physiotherapist, social workers, home care staff and administrators. The occupational therapist's main responsibilities are likely to include the following.

> - To assist in providing a service to clients, who may be disabled, elderly or recovering from illness, enabling them to live as independently as possible and, where appropriate, with care and dignity;
> - To act as a departmental professional adviser on matters relating to disability, liaising where necessary with individuals or groups of disabled people;
> - To take referrals and to deal with them appropriately; this may be in providing advice to disabled clients and/or their families. It may mean long-term involvement in casework and in co-ordinating services which will facilitate independent living;

- To visit disabled persons, to carry out assessments of their abilities, short-term and long-term needs, and to make recommendations accordingly;
- To make careful note of the abilities and difficulties which the carer(s) may be having. This has risen much higher on the national agenda with the implementation of Section 8(1) of the Disabled Persons' Act 1986, which places a duty on local authorities to take account of the abilities of carers;
- To carefully record and report at all stages. This is necessary in order to check progress and to ensure that proposed action is taken. Such supervision ensures that facts can be ascertained in the event of a query or dispute. In the event of staff changes, clear records facilitate a smooth changeover and reduce hassle for client and therapist. Where, as in the installation of major house adaptations, considerable financial implications may be involved, it is essential that details are accurately recorded and dated for a possible audit inspection;
- To set in motion and follow through such action as has been agreed by the client and, where necessary, by senior members of staff in a supervisory capacity;
- To record those needs which have been identified but which cannot immediately be met by existing services, and to draw this information to the attention of managers or members of other council departments, if it is considered that services for other clients may be improved.

Staff in many housing departments involve the occupational therapists and representatives from local disability groups in the planning, location and design of 'special' housing. Other council departments are likely to consult the occupational therapists to advise on the design and adaptation of buildings which are either owned by, or under the management of, the council.

REFERRALS

The terminology 'patient' which is used in hospital is no longer used once the person returns home and becomes a 'client' of their social services department in respect of their changed circumstances. A large proportion of clients are referred by general practitioners, district nurses, relatives, neighbours or home helps, or they may request assistance for themselves; a relatively small proportion are referred directly from hospital. The occupational therapist should have access to the client's general practitioner and should keep them informed of progress, or otherwise. Referrals are prioritized according to the level of risk (COT, 1994b).

ASSESSMENT

The importance of the assessment cannot be overemphasized (see Chapter 7). The majority of clients will be visited at home, but others may be visited prior to discharge. A visit to the patient's home by any members of the team should be sensitive to the lifestyle and wishes of the client. Listening and observations skills enable a rapport to be established between therapist and client and, where appropriate, with the clients' family, neighbour, home carer or significant other person.

Methods of recording an assessment must comply with Sections 3 and 4 of the Disabled Persons' Act 1986 to ensure accuracy of factual material and to ensure that observations and conclusions are well and logically supported.

Assessment for what?

Even the most carefully completed referral form will not necessarily prepare the therapist for what they will find on visiting. Because there are as many likely situations as there are clients, and perceptions between need and demand vary, it is only possible to set down some general principles, which the following exemplifies.

Example – referral for assessment of bathing

The most frequent request is for assistance with bathing. This may be translated as the client having practical difficulties due to physical impairment. Assuming that they have a bath, the difficulties may be as follows.

- The bath is too high, too low, or slippery.
- There is a need for strategically placed grab rails, bath seat, or non-slip mat.
- A method of lifting the client into and out of the bath is required.
- A different kind of bath, or a shower, is required.
- A downstairs bath/shower room is required, as the client can no longer climb stairs.

On visiting, the therapist will frequently find that the client is having difficulties with activities other than bathing, but assistance has been sought with this particular activity as the client wishes to bathe and is unable to do so.

Clues to the clients' problems may lie in the way they move, time taken getting to the door and opening it, the way in which they sit or stand and the condition of the house. First impressions are important, but should be weighed carefully when the client is interviewed. If, after some preliminary questioning, it is apparent that the client is having difficulties in several areas of daily activity, the therapist may proceed to make a more detailed assessment or make arrangements to call again at a more mutually convenient time. It may also be deemed necessary to consult with the client's general practitioner or a relative of the client who should be present during the assessment.

What actions to follow the assessment?

The client's difficulty may be resolved by the therapist demonstrating and teaching a new technique in the way that a particular action is carried out, or it may be that by re-arranging some household furniture, with the client's agreement, the therapist can enable the client to move more freely.

Where the solution lies in providing an aid or piece of equipment that will enable the client to achieve independence, the therapist will either arrange delivery and instruct the client in its safe use, or arrange for this to be carried out by a helper/assistant.

Local policies vary over what can be provided as essential aids, and those that are thought desirable but not essential. Charging policies also vary. Many local authorities lend aids and equipment free of charge, only recouping the cost if the client moves to another local authority. Some local authorities make charges for certain specified items within a particular range, by price or by type of aid. Increasingly, shops and mail order companies stock the more commonly requested items, and clients are encouraged to purchase from them with advice from suitably experienced therapy or nursing staff.

Joint Equipment Stores are also being commissioned. These may be managed jointly by social services, NHS and voluntary organizations. Alternatively, large suppliers of hospital or mobility equipment are being commissioned to run Joint Equipment Stores on their behalf, thus enabling therapy and nursing staff to select and issue equipment on loan and to arrange for its collection when it is no longer required by the client. Such stores must have clear criteria, guidelines and training for staff, covering record keeping (in case of litigation), cleaning and repair (COT, 1990c).

Clients should always be instructed in the safe use of the equipment, especially when it is complex, such as hoists. Retrieval of equipment is also important, particularly after the death of the user, when the continued presence of the item may distress the bereaved. Some equipment can be cleaned, overhauled and re-used; some have a single use and should be destroyed.

ADAPTATIONS

Where the disabled person can no longer function independently without making alterations to the building in which they reside, more complex solutions may be necessary. Adaptations include structural alterations which affect the fabric of the building. The ownership of the property is important, as it is necessary to obtain permission from the owner before any alterations are made.

Simple adaptations include such items as grab rails and stair rails, small ramps, alterations to individual steps, alterations to window catches, lowering or raising of shelves and installation of raised electric sockets. Such adaptations may be carried out by an approved local contractor or technician. Major adaptations include additional downstairs facilities, such as WCs, shower/bathrooms or bedroom extensions. These are deemed necessary where the client is no longer able to go upstairs and does not wish, or cannot afford, to move house. In these circumstances consideration may be given to the installation of a personal lift or a stair-lift (Morgan, 1994). Such major work must have the agreement of the family and/or other users of the home.

The process of getting work done will depend on such factors as type and size of adaptation. For example, a grab rail will probably be fitted by a technician employed by the local authority social services department, or by a local contractor who caters for minor works. Major adaptations will be managed by an architect or building surveyor, and estimates or tenders will be sought before the building work can be commenced.

The success of any adaptation is measured by how far it accommodates the needs of the disabled person, and their immediate family or carer, in timely improvement in their quality of life and independence. Important factors in achieving success will include the following.

- The skill and imagination of the occupational therapist in carrying out a thorough and detailed assessment of the needs of the client in the short and the long term, and translating these into a realistic set of proposals for action;

- Good rapport and communication between the occupational therapist and the client and family whilst they reach agreement on what is required;
- Skilled team work, led by the occupational therapist, by all concerned in the design preparation and building of the adaptation. The team will probably include an architect (preferably one who has some understanding of the specific needs of the disabled or elderly person), environmental health officer (where a Home Improvement Grant is being sought), planning officer, finance officer/adviser, builder and (in council property) a member of the Housing Department;
- Sufficient funds being available to finance the recommendations at each stage;
- Clear communications at all stages of the design and building;
- Adequate preparation, both physically and psychologically, for the disruption that will inevitably occur when building works commence.

THE EXTERNAL ENVIRONMENT

Once it is ensured that a client can live independently indoors, it is logical that they will wish to go out, visit friends and relatives, and go to shops, post office, library, pub and railway station. The occupational therapist will frequently be involved in the process of getting the highway engineers to have kerbs lowered at strategic crossing points, and ensure the provision of non-obstructive street furniture, access to public buildings and adequate public facilities.

Some local authorities have introduced policies to accommodate some of the environmental needs of disabled people. An increasing number of local authorities are appointing access officers, whose responsibility it is to ensure that the access requirements of the Chronically Sick and Disabled Persons Act 1970, the 1976 Amendment and the Disabled Persons Act 1981 are implemented, and that architects, builders and developers not only understand their responsibilities towards disabled persons but do all that they can to act upon the recommendations.

OTHER ACTIVITIES

Increasingly, occupational therapists are recruited to work in day centres and residential homes for older people, encouraging mobility, independence, dignity and a good quality of life (HMSO, 1989).

CONCLUSION

Occupational therapists have responded to the move to community care, but demand for their services universally exceeds supply. There are three particular areas of work with older people: rehabilitation within the hospital, wheelchair services and resettlement in the community. All involve detailed assessment and inclusion of the older person and carers in any plans. Independence may be achieved by equipment such as aids or adaptations to the home. The occupational therapist is in a unique position to provide expert advice on these issues. Success is measured by timely meeting of the needs of the disabled person and their immediate family or carer, and improvement in their quality of life and independence.

REFERENCES

Blom-Cooper, L. (1989) (Chairman) *Report of Commission of Inquiry – Occupational Therapy: An Emerging Profession in Health Care*, Duckworth, London.
Burnard, P. (1989) *Counselling Skills for Health Professionals*, Chapman & Hall, London.
COT (1990a) *Occupational Therapy Definition* (SSP 140), College of Occupational Therapists, London.
COT (1990b) *Statement on Supervision in Occupational Therapy* (SPP 150), College of Occupational Therapists, London.
COT (1990c) *Statement on Professional Negligence and Litigation* (SPP 135), College of Occupational Therapists, London.
COT (1994a) *A Report on Return to Practice After a Career Break*. College of Occupational Therapists, London.
COT (1994b) *Statement of Occupational Therapy Referral* (SPP 125a), College of Occupational Therapists, London.
COT (1995) *Standards, Policies and Procedures*, College of Occupational Therapists, London.
DLF (current edition) *Hamilton Index – Wheelchairs*, (continually updated) from Disabled Living Foundation, London.
Griffiths, D. and Wynne, D. (1991) *How to Push a Wheelchair*, Disabled Motorists Club (West Midlands), Unit 2a, Atcham Estate, Shrewsbury, SY4 4UG.
HMSO (1989) *Homes are for Living in*, HMSO, London.
Male, J. and Massie, B. (1990) *Choosing a Wheelchair*, Royal Association for Disability and Rehabilitation, London.
Morgan, J. (1994) *John's Guide* (Section K: Stairlifts), John Morgan, 12 Swan Road, West Drayton, Middlesex.
Please, P. (1990) *Able to Garden: A Practical Guide for Disabled and Elderly Gardeners*, Batsford, London.
SSI (1991) *Assessment Systems and Community Care*, Social Services Inspectorate, London.
Turner, A. (1992) *Occupational Therapy and Physical Dysfunction*, Churchill Livingstone, Edinburgh.

USEFUL ADDRESSES

The College of Occupational Therapists,
6–8 Marshalsea Road,
London SE1 1HL

Disabled Living Foundation,
380–384 Harrow Road,
London W9 2HU

Other essential services for rehabilitation of older people

15

The generally considered 'core' services for assessment and rehabilitation of older people have been described. There are also a number of other services which play an important role in certain circumstances. An understanding of the criteria for referral and their timely contribution will enable the core team to provide a truly comprehensive and effective rehabilitation service. Examples such as nutrition, dentistry, pharmacy, continence, hearing and optical services are described, and local developments may offer an even wider range. As will be seen from these contributions, the linkages and overlaps are considerable – but often overlooked. Good lateral working relationships between all members of the team will do much to facilitate a smooth and timely rehabilitation process. Smaller departments having episodic contact with the core team may feel isolated and excluded from its work and social activities, and opportunities for involvement should be actively pursued – and responded to.

Part a: Nutrition and dietetics in old age

Kiran Shukla

INTRODUCTION

Nutrition plays a key role in the health of an older person. Good nutrition for older people is important for both long-term and short-term health. The impact of illness and disability on nutritional status and the effects of this on the ability to recover from illness are of special concern in this age group. The ageing process affects the majority of the body systems including the gastrointestinal, cardiovascular, endocrine, renal, neurological, immune, sensory and skeletal systems. Along with these, social and financial circumstances may change. All these changes have a direct or indirect effect on nutritional status. Good nutrition is important not only for the maintenance of health, but also for the recovery from illness. This is particularly important for this age group, in which as a consequence of the natural ageing process ill health is more common.

The nutritional intake of older people relates closely to both physical and mental health. It also reflects on their social well being, but economic, psychosocial and physical factors also play a very important role in the general nutrition of this age group. There are no figures available for people with poor nutrition living at home, but it is well known that older people entering residential care are often malnourished. This could be because of long periods of poverty, illness, social isolation, or personal and psychological problems. It is very difficult for older people, especially from some ethnic minority groups, to accept that they cannot be looked after by the family any more. This can cause many psychological problems. Over the past decade, many changes have taken place in the provision of long-term care of older people.

A dietitian working in a dedicated unit for care of the older people or in the community needs a great deal of background information before appropriate advice is offered. This information can be as basic as the following.

- Is the patient at home or in residential care?
- If the patient is at home, who buys and cooks the food?
- Who delivers the food?
- How is the food delivered?
- What does the meal look like?
- Is the meal culturally/religiously acceptable?
- Can the patient handle crockery and cutlery?
- Will the patient get help in feeding?
- Are the meals rushed?
- If dentures are used, is the fitting right, and the dentures within the patient's reach?
- What is the nutritional value of the meal?
- How much food is eaten?
- Are likes and dislikes considered?

Only state registered dietitians can practise within the NHS. Many dietitians working with older people undertake further specialist training in this area.

REFERRAL TO THE DIETITIAN

Older adults can be referred to the dietitian if they are:

- diagnosed as needing a special/therapeutic diet;
- not eating a full mixed diet, e.g. liquids only;
- experiencing poor appetite or refusing food;
- unable to maintain body weight composition/biochemistry, due to poor oral intake;
- overweight.

Individual dietary advice is available for those referred to the service by a registered medical or dental practitioner. However, general nutrition or dietary advice may be given to groups of clients without the need for such referral (Dietitians Board Disciplinary Committee, 1994). Local arrangements should be made and agreed in order for there to be effective referral of elderly patients to the dietetic service.

Dietetic intervention starts by assessment.

ASSESSMENT

The dietitian assesses nutritional status by looking at:

- weight changes
- hydration
- dietary intake
- clinical condition
- social assessment, e.g. home circumstance and mental condition
- drug therapy
- biochemical profile/haematological measurements if available or needed.

ROLE OF THE STATE REGISTERED DIETITIAN AS PART OF THE MULTIDISCIPLINARY TEAM

After assessment, individual goals are agreed with the patient and/or carer, and the dietitian. The dietitian liaises with the appropriate people to ensure that the patient receives the prescribed dietary therapy. The patient/carer is educated on the modified or therapeutic diet and receives written information. The dietitian continues to assess the patient and review the therapeutic diet, evaluating dietary intervention, either directly or by advising others on an appropriate monitoring method. The dietitian provides information relevant to the needs of the patient and carers.

The role of the dietitian as part of the multidisciplinary team can include:

- acting as a resource to the healthcare team in providing expertise;
- devising simple nutritional assessment forms for the care staff to use;
- facilitating an optimum nutritional intake in all older adults;
- providing appropriate nutrition and/or therapeutic dietetic information in a relevant way for each client;
- providing support, including education, to health professionals and others involved in the care of the older adult;
- enabling carers to appreciate and act to ensure that patients receive nutritionally adequate food;
- training staff to look out for signs of malnutrition.

There are specific conditions in which dietitians can play a major role.

DYSPHAGIA

Here, close liaison with the speech and language therapist is very important. Multidisciplinary dysphagia groups can be very useful, to look at protocols for the treatment of the dysphagic patient. Dietitians can advise on appropriate nutrition, following the assessment of swallowing by the speech and language therapist in conjunction with the patient (see Chapter 9).

Appropriate thickeners for the food can be recommended by the dietitian. If it is decided to feed the patient enterally, the dietitian advises on the appropriate feed for the patient and the regime, which is regularly reviewed and monitored.

CONSTIPATION

Constipation is a common complaint particularly in immobile patients. Simple constipation can usually be prevented by increasing the intake of dietary fibre, of both cereal and vegetable origin, and by increasing the fluid intake.

The use of high-fibre diets is effective only if there is sufficient liquid to absorb the fibre and soften the stools. Some older adults may be reluctant to increase fibre, because of fear of pain or discomfort on defaecation. Older people should be advised to increase the fibre in the diet gradually by introducing new sources of fibre slowly over a few weeks. The body thus adjusts to the new diet more easily and the feeling of discomfort can be avoided.

The habit of sprinkling 'bran' over food should be discouraged, as it impairs the absorption of trace elements and minerals such as iron, calcium and zinc, along with affecting the palatability of the food. Dietitians can advise on the appropriate diet.

PREVENTION OF MALNUTRITION/PRESSURE SORES

The prime objective of nutrition policies and practices concerning the elderly should be directed towards the prevention of malnutrition. Those older people who are relatively inactive require fewer calories, because they use less energy. Although the energy requirement of such people may be lower, their requirements for other nutrients will not have changed and may well have increased. Their diet therefore should be one of quality rather than quantity. Wheelchair-bound or bedridden people are likely to put on weight because of immobility and are at general risk of pressure sores. It is advisable to consult the dietitian prior to putting patients on weight-reducing diets, which may not be nutritionally adequate.

APPROPRIATE DIET

Dietitians can ensure that adequate nutrition is not only given to the patient but is actually eaten by the patient. The nutritional value of the food not eaten is nil, hence the food served needs to be acceptable, palatable, of correct consistency and presentable to excite the patient's appetite. Over-zealous attempts to apply healthy eating guidelines to the elderly can result in nutritional problems. The overall message should be to keep up an interest in and enjoy the food. If the elderly could be encouraged to be more physically active, their energy requirements and their appetite would increase. Physical activity would also improve their body fitness and their general health and well being (see Chapter 8).

Some older people, especially those with infections (Lehmann, 1991; Mobartham and Trumbore, 1991; Sullivan, Walls and Lipschitz, 1991) may require a higher level of protein, but advice should always be sought from the dietitian and/or doctor on the level of protein required.

Whilst advising the carers, dietitians can give suggestions of appropriate foods, shopping on a budget for the client and information on stocking an accessible store cupboard for their clients. Here the dietitian can work very closely with other professionals and carers, to ensure that their advice is reinforced and is consistent.

THE FUTURE

Dietitians will also be involved in nutritional health promotion programmes in the hospital. They will identify areas for active promotion of health to patients/relatives and carers within the hospital. They will monitor the effects of health promotion, and will recognize the multidisciplinary role in promoting nutrition.

Dietitians have a vital role to play in the education and training of patient, caterers, nursing staff and other members involved in the care of the elderly. Training is also important for the social services staff involved in providing meals in the community.

REFERENCES

Lehmann, A.B. (1991) Nutrition in old age: an update and questions for future research, part 1. *Reviews in Clinical Gerontology*, 1, 135–45.

Mobartham, S. and Trumbore, L.S. (1991) Nutritional problems of the elderly. *Clinics in Geriatric Medicine*, 7(2), 191–214.

Sullivan, D.H., Walls, R.C. and Lipschitz, D.A. (1991) Protein energy undernutrition and the risk of mortality within 1 year of hospital discharge in a select population of geriatric rehabilitation patients. *American Journal of Clinical Nutrition*, 53, 599–605.

FURTHER READING

Department of Health (1993) *The Nutrition of Elderly People*, COMA Report No. 43, HMSO, London.

Nutrition Advisory Group for Elderly People (1993) *Dietetic Standards of Care for the Older Adult in Hospital*, British Dietetic Publication, Birmingham.

Thomas, B. (ed) (1994) *Manual of Dietetic Practice*, 2nd edn, Blackwell Scientific Publications, Oxford.

Part b: Dentistry and old age

Joyce Smith

THE PREVALENCE OF ORAL DISEASES

During the last quarter of a century, there has been a general improvement in oral health in many Western countries and this has resulted in more people keeping their natural teeth throughout life. In the United Kingdom, between 1968 and 1988 the proportion of older people with some natural teeth nearly doubled. Thus, in 1988, 43% of people aged 65–74 and 20% of those 75 and over were dentate. It is predicted that by the year 2038 the proportions will have risen to 85% and 81%, respectively (Todd and Lader, 1991). When the oral health of older people is considered, therefore, the prevalence, prevention and treatment of diseases of the natural dentition must be recognized as well as the problems associated with denture wearing.

Dental caries (decay) and periodontal (gum) diseases are the principal diseases of the oral cavity. In 1988, 45% of dentate people aged 55 and over in the United Kingdom suffered from dental decay and the majority (97%) had some form of periodontal disease (Todd and Lader, 1991). The nature of dental caries activity in older adults is different from that in the young, in that secondary, or recurrent, decay tends to predominate over primary lesions and caries of exposed tooth roots is particularly prevalent (Billings, Brown and Kaster, 1985).

Ill fitting dentures are very common in older people and a high prevalence of associated diseases of the oral mucosa has been reported (Smith and Sheilham, 1980; Todd and Lader, 1991). Carcinomas in and around the mouth must also be considered. These account for 1–4% of all malignant disease in the United Kingdom and amount to 1900 new cases and 950 deaths each year. Of cases of oral carcinoma, 85% occur in people over 50 years of age (Johnson and Warnakulasuriya, 1993).

All of these oral conditions may detract significantly from a person's general and social well being by causing pain and discomfort, problems with eating and speaking and prejudices associated with a poor appearance (Smith and Sheiham, 1979). It is important, therefore, that the oral health of older patients should be maintained during rehabilitation, in order that preventable, or treatable, conditions should not become added burdens for those whose health is already compromised.

ORAL SCREENING

Despite the high prevalence of oral disease in older people, there is a reluctance among many in this age group to seek dental care. Indeed, in the first quarter of 1995, only 33% of people aged 75 and over in England and Wales were registered with a dentist. Reasons for this low demand for care include fear, the cost of treatment, lack of mobility and the feeling that 'older people should not trouble the dentist' (Smith and Sheiham, 1980).

In many instances, chronic oral problems, which have been ignored by the patient, become acute and are brought to the attention of carers and members of the rehabilitation team at the time of a generally debilitating illness. In particular, patients may complain of pain, swellings, oral ulceration and loose dentures. It is essential that none of these symptoms should be ignored, but that arrangements should be made for a dentist to examine the patient as soon as possible either in a practice, or through a domiciliary visit. For new patients, carers and members of the rehabilitation team might find it helpful to complete a short checklist on oral symptoms in order to identify those in immediate need of dental care.

Because of the high level of oral pathology in older people, however, it is important that both those with natural teeth and those without should have regular oral examinations, whether or not they are experiencing symptoms. Oral screening allows for the identification and treatment of disease and for the implementation of appropriate preventive regimes. People should be encouraged to attend a general dental practice for routine check-ups, but where this is not possible, the examinations should be carried out on a domiciliary basis. In many districts, oral screening programmes are carried out in residential homes and hospitals. Clinical protocols should also provide for all older people admitted to hospital to receive an oral examination as part of the overall assessment of health.

PREVENTION OF ORAL DISEASE

During a debilitating illness a person's eating habits may alter and their ability to carry out adequate mouth care may be compromised. This may result in a poor level of oral hygiene and a marked deterioration in oral health. It is essential that carers and members of the rehabilitation team should be aware of this and help the patient to adopt good oral health practices. Where a patient is unable to maintain adequate oral self care, carers should be encouraged to assist with oral hygiene and provide balanced diets.

Dental decay occurs when bacterial plaque produces acid as a result of the metabolism of refined carbohydrates, especially sugars. The acid initially causes demineralization of the enamel surface, but caries and the breakdown of the tooth results if there are frequent acid attacks.

Limiting the frequency of consumption of sugary foods and drinks is, therefore, one of the most important ways of preventing dental decay. In particular, older people should be warned about sudden changes of diet. Constant 'snacking' on sugary foods and drinks instead of eating balanced meals should be discouraged, because of the risk of dental decay as well as from the general nutritional point of view.

Many older people suffer from dry mouth, xerostomia, and may be highly susceptible to dental caries, especially if they suck sweets, or take frequent sips of sugar-containing drinks to alleviate the symptoms. The dry mouth is usually due to the ageing process, or the patient's medication, but it should always be investigated, as it may be caused by an underlying systemic disease such as diabetes. If the dryness persists, safe alternatives such as sipping drinks with no added sugar, sucking sugar-free sweets, or the use of artificial saliva may be suggested. Sugary medicines are another potential cause of dental caries, particularly in people with a dry mouth, and should be replaced by tablets, capsules or sugar-free formulations wherever possible. As well as diet control, regular brushing with a fluoride toothpaste and the use of fluoride rinses are important measures for the prevention of dental decay. The fluoride increases the resistance of the enamel to acid attack and helps arrest early carious lesions.

Periodontal diseases affect the tissues supporting the teeth. The main cause is dental plaque, which initially produces inflammation, redness and bleeding of the gums. If the disease is not controlled at this stage it will progress to the underlying tissues; recession of the gums may occur and eventually the teeth will become mobile and may be lost. The older dentate patient should be encouraged, therefore, to maintain a level of oral hygiene which is adequate to prevent any further progression of periodontal disease. This may be carried out by regular brushing of the teeth, particularly near the gums, using a small-headed nylon toothbrush. For people who have difficulty holding a thin handle, an occupational therapist should be consulted for advice on toothbrushing aids. The toothbrush handle can be adapted to increase its size and allow it to be gripped more easily. Similarly, an electric toothbrush may prove beneficial for a patient with a weak grip. If a patient is suffering from severely bleeding gums, a chlorhexidine gel may be used to brush the teeth and gums until the situation has improved and then brushing should continue with a regular toothpaste. Carers should be encouraged to brush a patient's teeth if they are physically unable to do so. The carer should stand behind the patient and support the head under the chin with one hand whilst brushing the teeth with the other. If co-operation is difficult, extra help may be required and the patient may need a great deal of encouragement and reassurance. Initially it may only be possible to clean one or two front teeth until sufficient confidence is built up to brush all the dentition. The importance of oral hygiene for the older patient cannot be over-emphasized if the deterioration of extensively restored 'surviving' dentition is to be prevented.

Much of the pathology of the oral mucosa associated with denture wearing may be prevented by the correct care and maintenance of the dentures. Plaque and food debris should be removed regularly by brushing with soap and water and a small nylon brush. If this is carried out over a basin of water, breakages may be prevented. Persistent staining and hard deposits may be removed by the careful use of a proprietary cleaner. Dentures should be left out at night to allow the tissues to 'rest' and this, together with good denture hygiene, will help prevent denture stomatitis, a candida infection that may occur under dentures.

Carers should be aware that traumatic ulcers caused by ill fitting dentures may occur and can be resolved in most cases by leaving the dentures out and by arranging for a dental surgeon to modify the appliance. If necessary, the denture may be relined, or remade, at a later date. An ulcer that does not resolve after two weeks should always be investigated further, in case of malignancy.

Denture marking is another important preventive measure. Many older patients lose their dentures during the initial stages of a debilitating illness, particularly if they move between accommodations and have a series of different carers. This loss of dentures causes further problems at an already distressing time. Some dentures are marked when they are made, but where this has not been done, a denture marking kit may be used, or, as a temporary measure, the patient's name may be written on the smooth surface of the denture with a pencil and the lettering covered with clear nail varnish.

DENTAL TREATMENT

Dental treatment needs to be integrated into the overall plan for rehabilitation and should seek to alleviate any problems that might hinder the process. As many medical conditions may affect dental treatment, it is important for a dental surgeon to liaise closely with other members of the rehabilitation team.

The dentist will need to assess the patient's general and oral health and propose a realistic treatment plan in conjunction with the wishes of the patient and carers. The aim of the treatment should be to secure a standard of oral health that enables the patient to eat, speak and socialize without active disease, discomfort or embarrassment.

Initial treatment must seek to relieve pain and discomfort. For people with natural teeth, this may involve the stabilization of carious lesions and, in some cases, the extraction of grossly carious, or very mobile teeth, providing the treatment will not compromise the patient. Once this first phase has been completed, preventive care should be implemented as outlined above, together with a thorough scaling to remove gross deposits. Further treatment, including more complex restorative treatment, may be carried out at a later date when the patient is able to cope with longer treatment sessions.

Older people may have worn complete dentures for many years and be very skilled at controlling them. After a debilitating illness, however, the dentures may become loose for a variety of reasons including weight loss, a loss of muscle control following a stroke, or a dry mouth caused by medication. Initially, it is preferable to try and modify the existing dentures, as the older patient may not be able to adapt to a new set. In many instances the dentures may be adjusted and relined to improve their fit and make them 'tighter'. If this is not successful, new dentures, of a similar design to the old ones, may be made using a copying technique. For a person with a very dry mouth, where there is little retention of the dentures, consideration may be given to the use of artificial saliva. People whose dentures have been lost during their illness should have new dentures made as soon as they are able to cope with treatment. Where possible, photographs of the patient with natural teeth, or their previous dentures, should be consulted to aid in the construction of the new denture. It is crucial, however, that care staff should recognize the importance of keeping patients' dentures safely, in order that new appliances do not have to be made at a time when the patient is least able to adapt to them.

A number of alternatives exist for the delivery of dental care. Where a person is registered with a general dental practitioner, they should be encouraged to seek care from that dentist, either at a surgery, or on a domiciliary basis. Denture work, oral hygiene measures, and some simple fillings and extractions may all be carried out at home, or on a hospital ward. There is no reason, therefore, for the older patient to be unable to obtain treatment simply because they are unable to visit a surgery. Where a patient is unable to obtain treatment from a general dental practitioner, care may be provided by members of the community dental service, who have a special remit to provide care for people with disabilities. At the end of a course of treatment is is important to ensure that arrangements are made for future check-ups to monitor and help maintain the patient's oral health.

Good oral health is necessary for a person's general and social well being. It is important, therefore, that dental care should be recognized as an integral part of the rehabilitation of the older patient.

REFERENCES

Billings, R.J., Brown, L.R. and Kaster, A.G. (1985) Contemporary treatment strategies for root surface dental caries. *Gerodontics*, **1**, 20–7.

Johnson, N.W. and Warnakulasuriya, K.A.A.S. (1993) Epidemiology and aetiology of oral cancer in the United Kingdom. *Community Dental Health*, **10**(Suppl. 1), 13–29.

Smith, J.M. and Sheiham, A. (1979) How dental conditions handicap the elderly. *Community Dentistry and Oral Epidemiology*, 7, 305–10.

Smith, J.M. and Sheiham, A. (1980) Dental treatment needs and demands of an elderly population in England. *Community Dentistry and Oral Epidemiology*, **8**, 360–4.

Todd, J.E. and Lader, D. (1991) *Adult Dental Health 1988 – The United Kingdom*, HMSO, London.

Part c: Pharmaceutical care for the older patient

Alison Blenkinsopp

WHY IS PHARMACEUTICAL CARE NEEDED?

With the shift of emphasis from secondary to primary care in the NHS, and the philosophy of 'Care in the Community', more and more elderly patients will be treated at home.

The treatment of elderly patients often involves drug therapy. A patient may be admitted into hospital and be discharged on a complicated regime involving several drugs or have their admission medication totally changed. Multiple pathologies in elderly people often result in an array of drugs being prescribed. Strong communication and team work are needed if the key health professionals (GPs, community nurses, community pharmacists, dietitians and so on) are to achieve maximum benefit for the patient. In some cases this means establishing and building new links between professionals and including patients in the team.

Medication usage increases with age and many of those aged 65 years and over take several medicines. Research evidence has demonstrated the benefits of continuing drug treatments into old age. One example of how practice has changed in recent years is the treatment of high blood pressure (hypertension). Such treatment has been shown to be beneficial up to the age of 85 years in reducing ill health from heart disease and stroke (BMA/RPS, 1995).

While elderly patients are most likely to be taking different medications, they are also among the most vulnerable to potential problems. These include adverse reactions to drugs, interactions between drugs and difficulties in adhering to prescribed regimes (Figure 15).

In addition to (and sometimes instead of) prescribed medicines, patients also take non-prescription medicines, commonly known as over-the-counter medicines. Such medicines may be purchased from pharmacies or from other outlets such as drugstores and supermarkets. Commonly taken products include laxatives, painkillers and indigestion remedies.

We know that sometimes patients share medicines (both prescribed and over-the-counter drugs) or 'lend' them to others. This practice should be warned against at every opportunity, because of the potential for adverse drug reactions and interactions. Finding out who is taking what can sometimes be a difficult and complicated process.

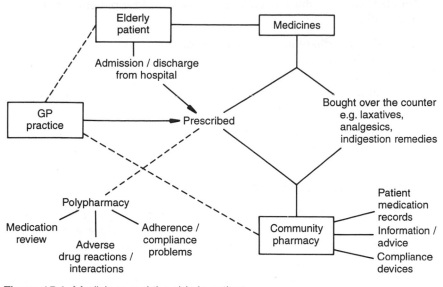

Figure 15.1 Medicines and the elderly patient.

There is clearly a need for collaboration between health and social care workers to help patients get the best from their medicines. Increasingly pharmacists' practice is moving towards pharmaceutical care, bringing with it a philosophy of team working. In addition the community pharmacist (the person who used to be known as the 'retail chemist') is asked for information and advice on a range of health and lifestyle matters including nutrition, smoking cessation, foot problems, incontinence and many others. Referral to and from other health professionals could be used more effectively to maximize the use of expertise.

WHAT IS PHARMACEUTICAL CARE?

The term 'pharmaceutical care' encompasses a philosophy of practice whereby the pharmacist works more closely together with patients and doctors (prescribers) (Canaday and Yarborough, 1994). The goals of pharmaceutical care are to achieve drug therapy that is effective in treating the condition(s) and to minimize problems such as side-effects. The term 'medicines management' is also relevant and describes actions to achieve effective drug therapy, in terms of therapeutic outcomes and best use of resources. Other healthcare workers, together with carers and relatives, have a key role in monitoring medicines in use.

The key issues in pharmaceutical care for the older patient are summarized as follows.

- Compliance/adherence with treatment;
- Adverse drug reactions (side-effects)
- Medication review;
- Physical sensory problems (failing eyesight, poor manual dexterity, memory loss, confusion).

Each of these issues will be addressed in turn, with suggestions of possible methods of problem resolution.

COMPLIANCE/ADHERENCE

'Compliance' in this context might be defined as the extent to which a person does/does not follow the instructions and take their medicines as intended by the prescriber. The term 'adherence' now tends to be used instead, since it is considered to be less judgemental/paternalistic. Primary non-compliance is where the patient does not have their prescription dispensed. Research suggests that this occurs with 15% of patients (Beardon, 1993). Secondary non-compliance is most common, where the patient has the prescription dispensed but does not adhere to the doctor's instructions. Research on factors influencing patients' adherence to prescribed medication has been extensive (Cramer et al., 1989; Larrat, Taubman and Willey, 1990; Donovan and Blake, 1992; Matsuyama, Mason and Jue, 1993), yet has failed to produce a coherent effective strategy for improvement. Variables including age, gender ethnicity and educational level have been explored.

More recent work has focused on patients' views and feelings about medicines and indicates that those with negative or mixed views about medication generally might be less likely to adhere to treatment (Britten, 1994). This behavioural approach may prove more fruitful in identifying possible strategies, because it is likely that patients' underlying beliefs and attitudes are the fundamental determinants of adherence.

Health professionals may believe that simply giving more information to patients will automatically bring about a change in behaviour. There is evidence that written 'reminder' charts can help (Raynor, Booth and Blenkinsopp, 1993). Patient information leaflets can also be valuable, providing careful attention is paid to the use of plain English and to the design, type size, and so on (Gibbs, Waters and George, 1990; Kitching, 1990; Raynor, 1992). Specific information about particular diseases and conditions can help to improve understanding (Cantrill and Cass, 1989; Dawes and Cantrill, 1990, Gibbs, Waters and George, 1990). Patients' interpretation of label instructions has been shown to vary (Holt et al., 1992) and it is helpful to reinforce the information.

Prescribers should be encouraged to state the exact dose on the prescription, even when the patient has had the medicine before, so that the label is explicit. Phrases such as 'to be taken as directed' or 'take as before' are unhelpful.

In many chronic conditions the patient will need to take medication for many years, yet perceived benefits may not be clear, unless troublesome symptoms are seen to be improved when the medication is taken.

ADVERSE DRUG REACTIONS (SIDE-EFFECTS)

In some cases, in which the condition itself is symptomless (e.g. hypertension) the drug therapy may make the patient feel worse through side-effects. Such circumstances mean patients' reluctance to adhere to the prescribed regimen becomes understandable.

An estimated 5% of hospital admissions are thought to occur as a result of adverse drug reactions. Particular drug groups are well known to be associated with problems in elderly patients:

- diuretics ('water tablets');
- non-steroidal anti-inflammatory drugs (used in rheumatic and arthritic conditions);
- hypnotics ('sleeping tablets').

Drug interactions sometimes occur when a drug is added to existing medication. Non-prescription drugs bought and taken by the patient can sometimes interact adversely with prescribed medicines.

Some drugs can cause or contribute to urinary incontinence (e.g. fast-acting diuretics). Others may cause constipation, occasionally resulting in overflow faecal incontinence.

MEDICATION REVIEW

Some 75% of prescribing by general practitioners is for repeat medication. Periodic review of medicines is an important mechanism for ensuring that inappropriate medicines or those which are no longer needed are stopped. Review should include monitoring for adverse drug reactions and drug interactions and identify any problems the patient is having with their medicines.

In the USA pharmacists working in the community (in retail pharmacy) are becoming increasingly involved in medication review. This trend is beginning to appear in the UK, where there are several pilot projects, looking at:

- review of nursing home residents' medication (Somerset);
- review of residential home residents' medication (Somerset);
- visits to patients in their own homes (Enfield, Haringey, Essex, Kirklees);
- follow-up of patients discharged from hospital.

FOLLOW-UP AFTER HOSPITAL DISCHARGE

During a stay in hospital, there are often changes to a patient's medication, with dosage alterations, addition of additional drugs and/or deletion of previous therapy. Unfortunately all sorts of problems can occur when the patient is discharged. Many hospitals now only give a few days' supply of medication for the patient to take home (7 days is increasingly common). Communication problems can result in a delay in the patients' GP being told by letter about medication changes. The importance of early discharge letters/faxes cannot be over-emphasized. Sending a copy of information about the medication to the patient's regular community pharmacy could be invaluable. This enables the pharmacist to have advance notice so that drugs can be ordered if necessary. The medicines can be delivered to the patients' home if necessary – many community pharmacists now provide this service. The pharmacist can liaise with the GP to ensure that repeat prescriptions are timely. Patients are sometimes not clear about what they should do with stocks of medicines they took previously. They may run out of supplies of their 'new' medicines and revert to taking what they have at home. They may even take both. Carers need to be alert to check medication after discharge from hospital. Talking with the local community pharmacist (who may have received a discharge checklist from the hospital pharmacist) can help to sort out any problems. Most community pharmacists now have computerized patient medication records (PMRs) and are in a good position to identify previous medication.

PHYSICAL/SENSORY PROBLEMS

More basic problems can sometimes occur. Simply getting the medicine container open can be a real struggle for some patients. Pharmacists routinely use child-resistant closures on all medicines now, to help reduce accidental poisoning in children, but will use ordinary caps on request. Special winged caps may be available to help those with arthritic hands – ask at the local pharmacy.

Loose tablets in bottles are becoming less common with the move towards individual patient packs. Foil and blister packs are common. Elderly patients need to be shown how to press tablets out of the latter type. This may seem obvious, but some patients try to push tablets out through the transparent plastic and give up when this cannot be done. Research suggests that elderly patients have more problems with blister packs compared to standard table bottles (Horner, Lochery and Sayegh, 1989).

Some pharmacy computers can produce large print for labels – ask if this facility is available at your local pharmacy. Braille labels are also available with standard medication instructions. Team members should ask local pharmacies to find out what facilities are available and could suggest that patients/carers do this too. Community authorities should also press for such change.

Reminder charts can be helpful if poor memory is a problem. Special dosage packs, e.g. Redidos and Dosett, are available where the day's or week's medicine doses are packed into small compartments by the patient or pharmacist. Research indicates that although these devices can be helpful, their existence is not widely known (Walker, Bellis and Jumani, 1990; Murray *et al.*, 1993). Ask at your local pharmacy to find out more about the different types available and their cost. At the moment they are not prescribable on the NHS, but many are simple to use and reasonably priced. Monitored dosage systems such as Nomad and Manrex are increasingly being used in the community, for example in sheltered housing complexes.

ADMINISTRATION OF MEDICINES

When an elderly patient has difficulty in remembering to take their medicines, or problems of sight or dexterity, the most practical approach is for someone else to administer them. This practice has gone on for years, with relatives, partners, carers and even home helps involved. Those involved in administering medicines can ask the pharmacist to clarify anything they are unsure about. Simple dosage charts can be useful, with a space to tick when a dose has been given. There is no reason why administering medicines in this way need cause problems. Most carers are conscientious and scrupulous in checking that the correct amount has been given. Many social services departments now contract with local pharmacists to provide basic training about medicines for care staff and this approach is to be encouraged.

NON-PRESCRIPTION (OVER-THE-COUNTER) MEDICINES

As more medicines are transferred from the POM (prescription-only medicines) category to P (pharmacy-only sale), a wider selection of treatments is becoming available over the counter. Some of the medicines that have been transferred in this way are shown in Table 15.1.

As it becomes possible for a more potent medicine to be purchased, it becomes even more important to encourage elderly people to check first before buying. If the same pharmacy is used, the pharmacist will be familiar with their prescribed medicines and will be able to check the patient medication record. In this way the possibility of interactions and adverse effects will be reduced.

Table 15.1 Over-the-counter (OTC) medicines previously available only on prescription

Drug name	Uses	OTC brands	Prescription brand
Ibuprofen	painkiller	Nurofen	Brufen
Cimetidine	heartburn/dyspepsia	Tagamet 100	Tagamet
Ranitidine	heartburn/dyspepsia	Zantac 75	Zantac
Famotidine	heartburn/dyspepsia	Pepcid AC	Pepcid
Miconazole	vaginal thrush	Femeron	Gyno-Daktarin
Clotrimazole	vaginal thrush	Canesten I	Canesten
Hydrocortisone	dermatitis, eczema	Hc45, Lanacort	Efcortelan
Hydrocortisone	mouth ulcers	Corlan pellets	Corlan
Aciclovir	cold sores	Zovirax cold sore cream	Zovirax

Elderly people have many needs relating to their medication. Improved communication between professionals providing health and social care can help to resolve medication problems. To get started, get to know the local community pharmacist(s) providing care for your patients; you have a common goal in pharmaceutical care.

WORKING TOGETHER

Legal requirements mean that the community pharmacist has to be physically present during the hours the pharmacy is open. The requirement applies to the supervision of dispensing and sales of 'Pharmacy Only' medicines. One of the results is that the pharmacists cannot easily leave their premises to attend meetings or visit patients, unless they have another pharmacist to cover for them. However, meeting in the pharmacy is always an option.

On the other hand, this means that the pharmacist is easily accessible and you are going to find them in the pharmacy readily. Why not make contact, especially if you have particular patient medication problems you need sorting out? Talk to the pharmacist about referring patients –

this is a two-way street. The pharmacist might refer a patient to the nurse, health visitor, chiropodist, dietitian, continence advisor, physiotherapist, occupational therapist or GP, where needed. You might refer patients to the pharmacist for more in-depth information about prescribed medicines, compliance problems or non-prescription medicine choices. Opening the communication channels could bring true team working closer to reality.

REFERENCES

Beardon, P.H.G., McGilchrist, MM., McKendrick, A.D., McDevitt, D.G. and MacDonald, T.M. (1993) Primary non-compliance with prescribed medication. *British Medical Journal*, **307**, 846–8.

BMA/RPS (1995) *British National Formulary*, Number 29, British Medical Association/Royal Pharmaceutical Society of Great Britain, London.

Britten, N. (1994) Patients' ideas about medicines: a qualitative study in a general practice population. *British Journal of General Practice*, **44**, 465–8.

Canaday, B.R. and Yarborough, P.D. (1994) Documenting pharmaceutical care: creating a standard. *Annals of Pharmacotherapy*, **28**, 1292–6.

Cantrill, J. and Cass, Y. (1989) Diabetic patients' knowledge of hypertension. *Pharmaceutical Journal*, **989** (Suppl. R22), 243.

Cramer, J.A. et al. (1989). How often is medication taken as prescribed? *Journal of the American Medical Association*, **261**, 3273–7.

Dawes, C. and Cantrill, J.A. (1990) An information booklet for patients with diabetes and hypertension. *Pharmaceutical Journal*, (Suppl.) **R26**, 245.

Donovan, J.L. and Blake, D.R. (1992) Patient non-compliance: deviance or reasoned decision-making? *Social Science and Medicine*, **34**, 507–13.

Gibbs, S., Waters, W.E. and George, C.F. (1990) Prescription information leaflets – a national survey. *Journal of the Royal Society of Medicine*, **83**, 292–7.

Holt, G.A. et al. (1992) Patient interpretation of label instructions. *American Pharmacy*, **NS32**, 242–6.

Horner, R., Lochery, P.M. and Sayegh, A. (1989) Is there a compliance problem with elderly people using blister packs? *Pharmaceutical Journal*, (Suppl.) **R26**, 243.

Kitching, J.B. (1990) Patient information leaflets – the state of the art. *Journal of the Royal Society of Medicine*, **83**, 298–300.

Larrat, E.P., Taubman A.H. and Willey, C. (1990) Compliance problems in the ambulatory population. *American Pharmacy*, **NS30**, 82–7.

Matsuyama, J.R. Mason, B.J. and Jue, S.G. (1993) Pharmacists' interventions using an electronic medication-event monitoring device. *Annals of Pharmacotherapy*, **27**, 851–4.

Murray, M.D., Bird, J.A., Manatunga, A.K. and Darnell, J.C. (1993) Medication compliance in elderly out-patients using twice-daily dosing and unit-of-use packaging. *Annals of Pharmacotherapy*, **27**, 616–21.

Raynor, D.K. (1992) Writing patient information – a pharmacists' guide. *Pharmaceutical Journal*, **249**, 180 2.

Raynor, D.K., Booth, T.G. and Blenkinsopp, A. (1993) Effects of computer-generated reminder charts on patients' compliance with drug regimens. *British*

Medical Journal, **306**, 1158–61.

Walker, R. Bellis, L. and Jumani, S. (1990) A community pharmacy-based study to assess demand for compliance devices. *Pharmaceutical Journal*, (Suppl.) **R25**, 245.

Part d: Continence promotion in old age

Jill Mantle

INTRODUCTION

Continence of urine and faeces is fundamental to quality of life and to the sociological, psychological and physical well being of the individual. Therefore, it deserves very high priority at every stage in the planning of an older patient's rehabilitation. The quality and reliability of continence frequently controls the balance between success or failure in rehabilitation, because it is of such crucial importance to morale and to social integration. Nothing demoralizes an older person or de-motivates them from physical activity and effort more than perceiving that they may disgrace themselves in company and are becoming 'like a baby again'. Incontinence of urine and/or faeces carries a social stigma and causes great discomfort, shame, depression and loss of self esteem, and is expensive. Frequently, it results in sufferers withdrawing from society and positively avoiding social contact (Grimby *et al.*, 1993). It predisposes to infections and bed sores. It also has adverse effects on carers which can result in the sufferer being ostracized, neglected or even abused. It has been suggested that incontinence is a major factor in patients and carers reaching crisis point, with consequent referral to residential care and its attendant cost implications (Continence Foundation, 1995).

Continence in a patient is an indicator of positive prognosis and should be actively promoted. Where continence is disturbed, the matter must be critically addressed. It is often the case for older patients that little or no specific attention is given to **the reason** for any continence problems or to whether there is a cure. It is assumed that such problems are due to age and therefore irremediable; sadly patients and their carers rarely challenge this assumption or expect improvement. Rehabilitation of the older patient has tended to concentrate on trying to regain and/or increase independence in such physical activities as eating, dressing and walking, while just containing or coping with urinary and faecal leakage, often in very unsatisfactory and undignified ways. However, the health and social care team will find patients very motivated to contribute ideas and co-operate in rehabilitation plans, which include aspects designed to overcome problems with continence.

The ability to be continent is a construct of many factors:

- the ability to recognize and react to the need to empty the bladder and/or bowel both day and night;
- the ability to store urine and faeces temporarily and 'to hold on' reliably and for long enough to select and reach an acceptable place to void without leakage;
- sufficient balance, mobility and strength to get to an appropriate place/position and manage clothing/aids, ideally without help;
- the ability to void effectively and attend to own hygiene;
- the ability to return to the status quo.

Independence in toiletting is priceless; needing the help of another is problematic in terms of convenience as well as psychologically. For example, most public toilet facilities are single sex, which excludes an accompanying spouse; some people find that voiding is inhibited by the presence of another; and the conventions of certain ethnic groups preclude one partner assisting the other in such intimate matters (Chapter 3).

Continence of urine and faeces is a largely unappreciated human faculty until things start to go wrong. Incontinence, defined as the involuntary loss of urine and/or faeces at inappropriate times and places, is not a disease but a symptom, indicating that there is some underlying problem. It takes very little to threaten and disturb continence and the cause of the leakage may have absolutely nothing directly to do with any disease process, but be due to anxiety, depression, not knowing where the toilet is, having to wait in a long queue for a vacant toilet or for a commode to be brought. Medication can precipitate incontinence, as may some food, and drinks containing caffeine, e.g. tea and coffee. The co-operation of all team members in identifying and addressing such matters in an informed and considered way is essential.

The most common causes of incontinence are:

- weak sphincteric and pelvic floor muscles, leading to urinary leakage with effort – called genuine stress incontinence;
- an overactive bladder that contracts and may empty without voluntary initiation or warning (often on movement) – called urge incontinence; urge and stress incontinence may occur together;
- difficulty in emptying the bladder, due to a blockage to the urethra, e.g. enlarged prostrate gland in men, resulting in a dribbling overflow incontinence;
- disorders of the nervous system, resulting in a variety of motor and sensory deficits in the control of bladder and bowel function, ranging from emptying without warning to difficulty in emptying;
- constipation and other bowel problems, e.g. mega-colon, impacted faeces (common in inactive and/or institutionalized elderly people);

- any hindrance to reaching the toilet, such as physical disability or frailty, stairs, heavy doors, pain, confusion and poor signposting.

Table 15.2 Prevalence of incontinence in older and institutionalized people

	Percentage incontinent
Urinary incontinence	
Women living at home, over 65	10–20
Men living at home over 60	7–10
Either sex living in an institution	
Residential home	25
Nursing home	40
Hospital – long-stay	50–70
Faecal incontinence	
Men and women at home	
65–84 years	3–5
85+ years	15
Men and women in an institution	
Residential home	10
Nursing home	30
Hospital – long-stay	60

(*Source*: Royal College of Physicians, 1995)

For some people the leakage is very mild and/or infrequent; for others it occurs often and/or is severe. The prevalence of incontinence tends to rise for adults with age and is more common in women (Table 15.2). With increasing life expectancy for both sexes, it becomes ever more important to educate and inform the public regarding continence from an early age; prevention is so much better than cure. People need to be encouraged to value continence and to seek investigation/explanation for any disturbance of their usual patterns. Many localities now have a specialist nurse Continence Advisor, and their role is being developed and refined (Rhodes and Parker, 1993). A substantial range of clinically effective treatments for most types of urinary and faecal incontinence is available and cure or significant improvement is usually possible, even for many older people. According to the Association for Continence Advice (1993), '*Continence for all should be the initial aim*' and 'Where this proves impossible the highest standards of care and management should enable social continence'. See also the Charter for Continence (Table 15.3).

The ultimate success or failure of a whole rehabilitation plan will be considerably influenced by the patient's continence status and potential.

Table 15.3 Charter for Continence

The Charter for Continence presents the specific needs and rights of people with bladder or bowel problems. It outlines the resources available and the standards of care that can be expected.

As a person with bladder or bowel problems you have the right to:

- Be treated with sensitivity and understanding.
- Become continent if achievable.
- Receive a thorough individual assessment of your condition by a doctor or nurse knowledgable in this aspect of care.
- Request specialist advice about continence care.
- Be provided with a clear explanation of your diagnosis.
- Participate in a full discussion of treatment options, their advantages and disadvantages.
- Be provided with full, impartial information on the range of products which are available and how to obtain them.
- Expect products to have clear instructions for use.
- Receive regular reviews of treatment and be given the opportunity to change treatments if your condition has changed.
- Be made aware of any treatments or products as they become available.
- Be provided with a personal contact point able to give you on-going advice and support.

Developed by:

The Continence Foundation, InconTact, Association for Continence Advice (ACA), the RCN Continence Care Forum, the Enuresis Resource and Information Centre (ERIC), the Spinal Injuries Association and the Multiple Sclerosis Society.

Produced by an educational grant from Bard Limited.

March 1995

Therefore, relevant staff (especially nurses, physiotherapists and occupational therapists) must be thoroughly knowledgeable regarding the possible effects on continence of certain pathologies, medicaments and changes in environment. There should be corporate responsibility within the rehabilitation team for anticipating and avoiding problems where possible, or at least recognizing difficulties speedily. Key primary healthcare team members need to be trained to make an initial continence assessment to an agreed basic format as an integrated component of the holistic consideration of the patient's rehabilitation needs. Where necessary this assessment should then form the entry point to an efficiently managed, comprehensive specialist continence service (Table 15.4) which the Government has indicated should be the norm for every locality (DHSS, 1991; Association for Continence Advice, 1993). Components and models for such a service are discussed by the Royal College of Physicians (1995).

Table 15.4 Recommendations of the Royal College of Physicians (1995) on the components of a continence service

- a defined method of entry for patients referred by general practitioners, nurses, hospital staff and patients themselves
- access to appropriate diagnostic facilities, including urodynamic and anorectal investigations
- access to medical and surgical consultants with a special interest in incontinence
- integration of incontinence services for children with other paediatric services
- attention to the wishes of patients and carers
- access to nurses and physiotherapists with special training in treatment modalities for incontinence
- a role for one or more specialist continence advisors in the education of the public and professionals in continence maintenance
- a policy concerning the purchasing and supply of containment materials and equipment in the community, in residential and nursing homes and in hospitals
- well defined audit and quality assurance systems.

The structure required to achieve these aims might include: a designated manager, an expert advisory panel and a budget to provide staff, their training and support services, and containment materials and equipment.

ASSESSMENT BY THE PRIMARY HEALTHCARE TEAM

First-line assessments should be to standardized, evidence-based protocols agreed with their local continence service (Continence Foundation, 1995).

The assessment should include:

- careful, empathetic and unhurried enquiry into the exact history and nature of the problem from the patient and carers. There may be total denial of there being any problem. Social and environmental factors should be included;
- some form of 'round the clock' diary, e.g. frequency/volume charts, that record the time, frequency and volume of both intake (food and drink) and normal voiding (urinary and faecal) as well as episodes of incontinence;
- physical examination where appropriate, e.g. to identify prostatic outflow obstruction or faecal impaction;
- urine (ideally mid-stream) and blood tests, where indicated.

In the past, there has been a failure on the part of healthcare professionals (particularly in hospitals and residential care) to consider the normal taboos of society in relation to toiletting. For some individuals, a unisex toilet, toilets without doors, voiding in company, or no realistic means of washing and drying hands may be sufficient to inhibit voluntary voiding. Some women have been brought up never to sit on the toilet seat when voiding, except in their own home, for fear of infection; crouching to void predisposes to residual urine and infection (Moore and

Richmond, 1989). Others have a horror of sharing the use of a toilet with a stranger or of using a soiled toilet. Those readers who think this unduly fastidious would do well to reflect on the reasons for professional staff toilets invariably being separate from those for patients.

Great empathy, sensitivity and superior communication skills are required when listening and enquiring about continence problems from patients and/or carers. How this is done and the language used often determines whether the outcome is positive or negative.

There is always a danger that well informed health professionals, particularly in the community setting, will assume their clients have already tried all the simple remedies; for example simply drinking sufficient and eating appropriately to avoid constipation and ensuing faecal impaction induced by inactivity. Have they realized that some medications cause 'slow transmit time' as a side-effect or that malnourishment may result in reduced strength, so affecting manoeuvrability? Helping both patient and carer to understand their problems can be very helpful.

The objective of such an assessment is to form a clear picture and establish a working diagnosis that allows immediate remedial action to be taken and/or identifies those sufferers who require referral. According to the Continence Foundation (1995), 'There will be very few instances when provision of products is the only intervention indicated', and 'Referral criteria, and specification of who can refer, should be developed locally'. In addition, there should be clearly defined criteria for re-assessment, review and discharge. For example, where certain interventions have been tried but have failed to produce significant improvement in 8–12 weeks, referral to the continence service should be reconsidered.

TREATMENT

Treatment options include adjustments to fluid intake, diet and current medication; rehabilitation of the patient's strength and mobility; pelvic floor muscle re-education with or without biofeedback or neuromuscular electrical stimulation; bladder retraining; pharmacological agents; intermittent catherization and surgery. Once again, first line symptomatic treatment protocols are best set in consultation with the local continence service.

The basic principles are as follows.

- Treat infections.
- Attend to constipation/faecal impaction.
- Maximize patients' strength and mobility by means of graded activity and nourishing diet.
- Facilitate independence with mobility aids, easy clothing, grab rails and reasonable proximity to a toilet.

- Pelvic floor muscle re-education is appropriate for the sphincteric and pelvic floor weakness of mild to moderate genuine stress incontinence. Surgery should be considered for severe cases.
- Use anti-cholinergic agents, pelvic floor muscle contractions and bladder retraining for urgency and urge incontinence.
- Consider surgery to correct enlargement of the prostate.

Where possible, several alternative solutions should be suggested for continence problems to allow for the individual and carer to choose according to their perception of what is or is not acceptable and manageable. The whole issue needs discussing in some detail and, where appropriate the occupational therapist, physiotherapist and/or nurse continence advisor should be involved. For example, a commode may be acceptable, to save struggling all the way to the toilet, but the prospect of opening one's bowels on one sited in the sitting room may not be. Such feelings may be overcome or may prove strong enough to inhibit defaecation and cause constipation. Occasionally quite radical options may be worthy of consideration; for example, for the heavily dependent patient it may be reasonable to consider a catheter, for the carer's sake, even where urinary continence is substantially intact. As is described earlier in this chapter, expert dietary advice is available within the NHS and this should be called upon more readily.

MANAGEMENT OF INTRACTABLE INCONTINENCE

The objective of such management is to gain 'social continence', i.e. to organize or contain voiding in a way that is acceptable and practical to the patient and anyone else who has to be involved. It should also enable the patient to live life as fully as they are able and interact socially without fear of embarrassment, accidents or odour. Each patient's sensitivities must be accommodated and their dignity preserved as far as is humanly possible.

PRODUCT PROVISION

There is an increasingly wide range of products available, including disposable and re-usable bedding, pads and body garments, and collecting devices, e.g. penile sheaths, catheters and drainage bags; however, quality and price vary. As yet very little independent, scientific evaluation of products has been conducted and in addition patients have individual needs and preferences. As the patients become better informed there will be an increasing demand for choice. Supplies should be provided only after assessment by a designated and appropriately trained member of the continence service. The availability of over-the-counter products allows the assessment route to be circumvented, but denies the opportunity of treatment. The following factors have to be considered in collaboration with the patient and carer: the choice of the product(s) that are most appropriate; delivery or collection of supplies; storage of supplies; hygienic disposal of disposable products; laundry of soiled clothing, bedding and re-usable products; regular re-assessment and monitoring of patient needs and satisfaction.

The cost of product provision and allied services needed to support a patient with long-term incontinence is borne by the relevant health authority, except for private (paying) patients in hospitals and residential care. However, each health authority has discretion regarding eligibility as well as type, quality and quantity of products to be provided. There is also variation between authorities as to whether and by whom products are delivered or must be collected, and the arrangements regarding disposal and laundry.

Professionals, patients and carers who experience difficulty in obtaining help, information and/or advice on any continence matter should contact the Continence Foundation. It was established in 1992 with three key purposes – information, education and research. It has produced an excellent Continence Pack (Continence Foundation, 1992), and has up-to-date databases on facilities, specialist referral centres and continence aids. It organizes seminars and study days, contributes to a wide range of national initiatives to inform and raise awareness, and has a telephone helpline for the public and professionals: 9 am–6 pm on 0191–213 0050.

REFERENCES

Association for Continence Advice (1993) *Guidelines for Continence Care*, obtainable from ACA, Basement, 2 Doughty Street, London WC1N 2PH.

Continence Foundation (1992) *Continence Foundation Pack*, obtainable from The Continence Foundation, Basement, 2 Doughty Street, London WC1N 2PH.

Continence Foundation (1995) *Commissioning Comprehensive Continence Services: Guidance for Purchasers*, obtainable from the Continence Foundation, Basement, 2 Doughty Street, London WC1N 2PH.

DHSS (1991) *Agenda for Action in Continence*, Department of Health, London.

Grimby, A., Milson, I., Molander, U., Wiklund, I. and Ekeland, P. (1993) The influence of urinary incontinence on the quality of life of elderly women. *Age and Ageing*, **22**, 88–9.

Moore, K.H. and Richmond, D. (1989) Crouching over the toilet seat: prevalence, and effect on micturition. *Neurourology and Urodynamics*, 8(4), 422–4.

Rhodes, P. and Parker, G. (1993) *The Role of Continence Advisers in England and Wales*, Social Policy Research Unit, York.

Royal College of Physicians (1995) *Incontinence: Causes, Management and Provision of Services*, Report of a working party, Royal College of Physicians, London.

FURTHER READING

Bennett, G.C.J. and Ebrahim, S. (1995) *The Essentials of Health Care in Old Age*, 2nd edn, Edward Arnold, London.

Chiarelli, P. (1992) *Women's Waterworks*, Neen Health Books.

Chiarelli, P. and Markwell, S. (1992) *Let's Get Things Moving*, Neen Health Books.

Polden, M. and Mantle, J. (1990) *Physiotherapy in Obstetrics and Gynaecology*, Butterworth Heinemann, Oxford.

Sanderson, J. (1991) *An Agenda for Action on Continence Services*, Community Services Division, Department of Health, London.

Tobin, G.W. (1992) *Incontinence in the Elderly*, Edward Arnold, London.

Part e: Sight in old age: an orthoptist's contribution to rehabilitation

Janet Pierce

The orthoptic profession expanded during World War II, when it was found that R.A.F. pilots were struggling to maintain normal eye movements under the stressful conditions of night flying. Since then, orthoptists have taken over much of the therapeutic work which had previously been carried out by ophthalmologists. The orthoptist is trained to investigate, diagnose and treat abnormalities of sight, eye muscle movement and stereovision and is now increasingly involved in visual field assessment.

THE EYE AND AGE

It is well documented that the incidence of eye disease increases with age (Figure 15.2) and these changes are usually gradual and may not be identified by either the individual or those around them. If visual impairment is left undiscovered and untreated, it can cause a severe handicap, especially if accompanied by hearing defects, communication problems and physical disability (DLF, 1979). The visually impaired elderly person has been shown to become more isolated and withdrawn from society than those who have normal vision.

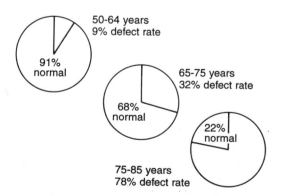

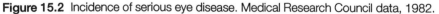

Figure 15.2 Incidence of serious eye disease. Medical Research Council data, 1982.

The current information-driven society is resulting in a plethora of written information about services available, criteria for access, quality standards and appointment schedules. Community-based care requires older people to take responsibility for such things as medication (see above section on Pharmaceutical care). The inability of older people to read this information will reduce its accessibility. Appropriate alternatives should be available. Authors of such information should note the need for large print and suitable colours and consider how the needs of those with the poorest vision can be met, for example through use of talking newspapers, etc.

As more people are living into their 80s, every attempt must be made to help older people maintain their independence. This includes making the maximum use of their vision whatever it may be to ensure safety, aiding daily living and the highest quality of life. In a survey of 161 patients who were regularly attending the physiotherapy and occupational therapy departments, it was found that 25% were functioning with gross visual deficit (Pierce, 1981). The ages of the patients ranged between 18 and 88 years, but 28 of this group were over 65 years and 12 of them had such poor sight that they could have been registered as blind. These were patients undergoing ADL training in kitchens, or learning to walk again – yet therapists and doctors were unaware of the baseline vision, which had not been included in any of the assessment procedures.

TREATMENT PLANS

The insidious development of poor vision puts the onus on the individual to make the necessary arrangements for improvement. Unfortunately many older people, their relatives and health professionals accept failing sight as irremediable and an accompaniment of old age. Many older people only need glasses prescribed to bring their eyesight to a level to allow them to live independently – to read their mail, cross the road, undertake personal care, etc. A visit to a high-street optician is needed and opticians are able to undertake home visits for those with mobility problems. If the individual is on a low income, the cost of the test and the glasses can be supplemented. Despite the relative ease of access to the services of an optician, surveys show that a large percentage of the population are using glasses that are out of date, and this percentage rises with age. In a specific study of one day-hospital undertaken by the author, 51% of those referred to an optician needed new or modified glasses. 'Sharing' glasses within families, and amongst groups of old people is well known, and the practice should not be encouraged by their informal or formal carers. The suitability and cleanliness of the lenses and the general state of repair of the glasses are both important to maximize vision. Inadequate home lighting is a further cause of impairment (Cullinan *et al.*, 1979) and its improvement will further facilitate vision.

SPECIFIC PROBLEMS

DOUBLE VISION

If there is diplopia (double vision) present its aetiology must be determined, but at the same time the orthoptist can help the patient with temporary relieving prisms that can be altered as the condition changes. The use of prisms, rather than the covering of one eye to remove double vision, will allow stereovision to be maintained, particularly important for depth perception, especially when walking, sitting, pouring liquids, etc. Eye exercises can also be given to relieve the patient's symptoms. If there is thought to be a disease of the eye then the patient should be referred to the ophthalmologist in the local eye department by the optician, the orthoptist or the GP.

CATARACT

Cataract extractions are now frequently performed by ophthalmic surgeons. The lens that has become opaque as a result of normal ageing is replaced by an implant. This results in normal vision with the help of a small correction with glasses.

GLAUCOMA

Glaucoma is a chronic eye disease most prevalent from the age of 45 years and caused by increased pressure within the eye, resulting in progressive loss of field.

DIABETES

Diabetes and macular degeneration are the diseases that are not easily treated and these are the main causes of low sight today (WHO, 1973). Patches of retina are damaged and cannot be repaired, resulting in loss of sight when fixing straight ahead, but peripheral areas remain intact.

REGISTRATION AS BLIND OR PARTIALLY SIGHTED

When eyesight cannot be restored then registration as blind or part-sighted can be advantageous to the older person and is set in motion by registration on a BD8 form by an ophthalmologist. It may give them priority for home helps or care assistants, especially if this is in addition to another disability. An appointment with the local Low Visual Aid clinic can introduce anyone to magnifiers and telescopes, and for those registered the Royal National Institute for the Blind (RNIB) advisor can make home visits for a more comprehensive assessment of equipment needs.

Few 'blind' people are without sight of some sort. It may be sight within a small area, but this might be good enough to read the bottom line of the letter chart. Such people would be registered as blind, not because of their vision, but because of their lack of field. The absence of field when looking down is more of a handicap to older people than the absence of the elevated field, due to their need to look out for barriers to mobility such as steps and obstacles. Loss of central vision is worse still, as the object under observation disappears as the eye attempts to focus. The definition of blindness (HMSO, 1990) is 'that a person should be so blind as to be unable to perform work for which the eyesight is essential'. This was defined with a working rather than ageing population in mind and excludes the normal daily living needs. If normal vision and a normal field remains in only one eye, then the patient can function fairly safely and cannot be classified as part-sighted. Initial problems with depth appreciation can be overcome in different ways over time. Part-sighted patients are those not falling into the blind definition, but they must be 'substantially and permanently handicapped by defective vision'. They are not eligible for the financial allowances of the blind, but with the help of the social services they can gain access to talking newspapers, large print books, concessionary fares, etc. The facilities will vary between local authorities within the UK, the aim being to improve their quality of life.

TIPS FOR THE MULTIDISCIPLINARY TEAM

The multidisciplinary assessment of older people should include the following:

1. Vision (for near and distance, using appropriate glasses);
2. Presence of a known eye problem;
3. Need for regular instillation of eye drops;
4. Date of last eye test/glasses;
5. Whether the glasses are the patient's own, and when were they prescribed.

Advice to patients by any member of the team should include:

1. Use of 100 watt light bulbs in all living areas in home;
2. Use of 60 watt reading lamp for close work;

3. Use of reading glasses for all close activities;
4. Use of distance glasses at other times.

Patients who should be referred on for specialist assessment (Figure 15.3) include those:

1. Identified through the initial assessments described above
2. Showing signs of or complaining of visual difficulty (can you get eye to eye contact?)
3. With an unusual head posture
4. Who close one eye intermittently
5. Who take little interest in their surroundings
6. With intermittent lack of confidence relating to stairs, pouring liquids, etc.

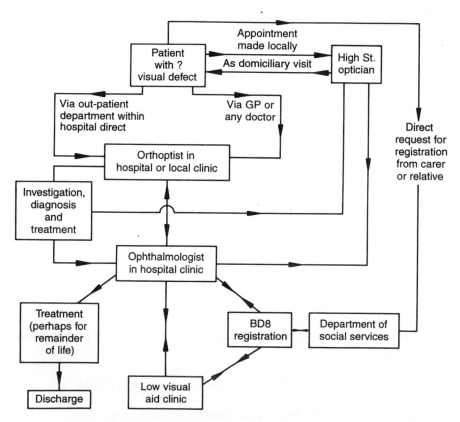

Figure 15.3 Possible referral patterns for a patient.

REFERENCES

Cullinan, T.R., Silver, J.H. *et al.* (1979) Visual disability and home lighting. *The Lancet*, **March**, 642–4.

DLF (1979) *The Elderly Person with Failing Vision*, Disabled Living Foundation, London.

HMSO (1990) *BD 8 Registration Form (Revised 1990)*, HMSO, London.

Pierce, J.M. (1981) Visual screening in rehabilitation depts. *Journal of Occupational Therapy*, **May**, 151–2.

WHO (1973) *The Prevention of Blindness*, WHO technical report series No. 518, World Health Organization, Geneva.

USEFUL ADDRESSES

Royal National Institute for the Blind (RNIB),
224 Great Portland Street,
London W1N 6AA

International Glaucoma Association (IGA),
Ophthalmology Department,
Kings College Hospital,
Denmark Hill,
London SE5 9RS

British Diabetic Association (BDA),
10 Queen Anne Street,
London W1M 0BD

Tapes for information: *Your Cataract Explained* and *Your Guide to Glaucoma*.
Information from
Eye Sister,
Charles Cookson Clinic,
Gloucester Royal NHS Trust,
Gloucester GL1 3NN

Booklet FB19 (1994) *A Guide for Blind and Part Sighted People*
from local DSS office.

Part f: Hearing in old age – audiology and hearing therapy

Jane Milligan and Fiona Watts

INTRODUCTION

A number of recent studies have demonstrated that hearing loss has an adverse effect on functional status, quality of life, cognitive function and emotional, behavioural and social well being (Uhlmann *et al.*, 1989; Mulrow *et al.*, 1990; Bess, Lichtenstein and Logan, 1991) (Figure 15.4).

Hearing loss
Psychological costs

1. Decreased self-esteem
2. Loss of independence
3. Depressed effect
4. Reduced enjoyment of leisure activities

Social costs

1. Avoidance of previously enjoyed activities
2. Inappropriate responses during conversations
3. Difficulty communicating over the telephone
4. Personal safety jeopardized by inability to hear warning signals
5. Inability to function with maximal efficiency at work

Figure 15.4 Potential psychological and social costs associated with unremediated handicapping. From Alpiner and McCarthy (1993), with permission.

Data are also beginning to accumulate documenting a link between hearing loss and cognitive status in persons diagnosed with dementia (see Chapter 8).

1. Hearing loss is more prevalent in older adults with dementia (Weinstein and Amsell, 1986).
2. Older adults with dementia are likely to have more severe hearing loss than those without dementia (Weinstein and Amsell, 1986, Uhlmann *et al.*, 1989).
3. The risk of dementia increases as a function of increasing hearing loss after adjustments are made for potentially confounding variables such as depression, primary prescriptions and age (Uhlmann *et al.*, 1989).

4. Unremediated hearing loss lowers performance on aurally administered diagnostic tests used to quantify the severity of senile dementia
   (Weinstein and Amsell, 1986).
5. Hearing aids lower scores on tests of cognitive function, suggesting improved mental status with hearing aid use (Mulrow *et al.*,
   1990).

HEARING CHANGES IN NORMAL AGEING

The term usually applied to the type of deafness associated with the ageing process is presbyacusis. This type of deafness is a progressive sensory
neural deafness that comes on and advances for no apparent reason with
the years.

It is due to an atrophy of the hair cells and auditory nerve fibres in the
cochlea, and is most commonly noticed around the age of 60, but a
premature onset may be associated with bouts of otitis media in childhood and particularly with prolonged exposure to noise throughout a
working life. We know very little about presbyacusis beyond the facts
that it is progressive; it is sometimes, but not always, associated with
high blood pressure or general atherosclerosis; high tones are affected
first and foremost and hearing by bone conduction is reduced, often
grossly so.

The singing of birds and the ringing of bells are lost first, but speech is
also difficult to follow, especially when it is rapid. Group conversation
becomes impossible, particularly in noisy surroundings, and general
slowing of the central reaction time makes matters no easier.

HEARING SERVICES

The traditional method of referral of adults with hearing loss is to the ear,
nose and throat (ENT) department, where the person will see a doctor
who takes a medical history and examines the ears (Figure 15.5). Hearing
will also be tested by an audiology technician and if necessary a recommendation will be made for a hearing aid to be fitted.

An alternative direct referral system may exist whereby the GP
can refer directly to the audiology service when a hearing aid is felt to
be the solution to the hearing problem. The primary aim of this method
of referral that by-passes the ENT department is removal of a significant proportion of patients from ENT waiting lists. GPs are
expected to ensure that such patients show no sign of significant ear
abnormalities. An audiological technician examines the patients using
a set of guidelines to identify potential medical conditions. Those who

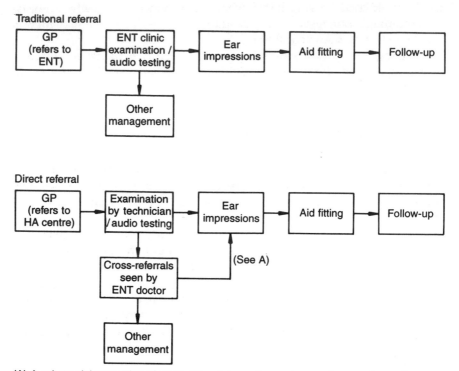

Traditional referral

Direct referral

(A) A substantial proportion of cross-referrals have the ear impressions, and sometimes fitting, before seeing the ENT doctor

Figure 15.5 Flow diagram showing principal routes of hearing aid provision followed by traditionally and directly referred patients. ENT, ear, nose and throat department; HA, hearing aid. From HMSO (1994), with permission.

indicate a medical need are cross-referred to the ENT department (Figure 15.5).

When a hearing aid is confirmed as the best solution, there will usually be at least three appointments at the hearing services centre.

1. An impression is taken of the ear(s), so that an individual ear mould can be made.
2. When the ear mould is returned from the manufacturer, a second appointment is made to fit the hearing aid. Explanation on how to use the aid to its best effect will be given.
3. Several weeks later a review appointment is offered to check on progress.

NHS hearing aid users can access a free battery and maintenance service from their local audiology department.

HEARING THERAPY

The hearing therapy service offers an aural rehabilitation service. Referral is usually made following hearing aid provision. The therapist will assess the patient's need and develop an appropriate therapy programme which may include:

- help with hearing and/or using hearing aids more effectively;
- improving communication skills;
- advice and information about aids to daily living such as TV and telephone adapters;
- advice and practical help with tinnitus;
- management of hearing-related balance disorders;
- counselling related to adjustment to hearing loss;
- help when communication difficulties exist with carers and/or families as a result of hearing loss.

Hearing therapists are usually found working alongside audiology departments and may operate an open referral system. They should also have close contact with speech and language therapists, occupational therapists, physiotherapists and clinical psychologists, for two-way access to relevant skills.

IMPROVED SETTINGS

Hearing loss affects individuals as well as their family, friends and colleagues. Information about how to help the person compensate for their impaired hearing needs to be shared as openly as possible. Jack Ashley, the deaf MP, wrote of the embarrassed confusion he saw on other people's faces when he first lost his hearing. Embarrassment stops many ordinary people from communicating with those who have disabilities. Sharing information can be very helpful in reducing this problem.

HOW THE TEAM CAN HELP

There are many ways in which the way we speak to someone who has a hearing loss will influence their ability to communicate with us. The following guidelines are appropriate whether or not a person uses a hearing aid. However, if the person does wear a hearing aid, remember it will function best at a distance of three to six feet.

1. Make sure the person is wearing their hearing aid if they have one. Also check that ears are clear of wax, and that the aid is switched on at the correct volume and has batteries that work.
2. Try to ensure that the person is facing you and that you have their attention before you begin to speak.
3. Keep background noise to the minimum possible. Noisy places such as busy clinics and large waiting rooms will always be more difficult. Do what you can to reduce background noise in your own environment.
4. Look at the person and do not turn away while you are talking to them.
5. Sit so that your face is well lit and not in shadow.
6. Your face and mouth are particularly important. Many people cover them with their hands without realizing it, especially when they are feeling uncomfortable. Try to allow the hearing impaired person to see your mouth as you speak.
7. Slow down slightly, but keep the rhythm or normal pattern of speech. This makes it easier to follow what is being said.
8. DO NOT SHOUT.
9. Use your facial expressions, body language and gestures to back up and clarify your speech. Unnecessary hand and head movements will distract, but appropriate non-verbal messages will complement the spoken word.
10. Find out if the person uses Makaton (a total communication system using signs and/or symbols and always supported by speech). If so then you should use it too.
11. If necessary repeat, or better, rephrase a sentence which has not been heard or understood. As a last resort you may want to write it down in words or symbols to help the person.
12. Give the person plenty of time to communicate. Be patient!

Patients regularly attending clinics who are known to have a hearing difficulty should have their case notes marked appropriately to ensure that relevant arrangements are made for calling them.

HOW THE ENVIRONMENT CAN HELP

A good acoustic setting is one with smaller dimensions, soft furnishings and good lighting. For example, a lounge will be an easier setting for someone than an open clinic or treatment area. This is because echoes and distortions are reduced.

The fewer people present, the easier it is to follow events. If a room is unavoidably crowded the person with a hearing impairment will find communication easier if they stand or sit with their back to a wall. Sound approaches them from fewer directions, so they can identify its source more easily.

Finally, there are some very simple ways to improve a poor acoustic setting. A tablecloth on a hard table, carpet on a hard floor, double glazing and/or curtains at a window, a tissue between cup and saucer will all help to dampen sounds. It is worth looking around to see if such measures can be taken in difficult settings.

ADDITIONAL TECHNOLOGY

There are many additional pieces of equipment to help people who have hearing impairment by alerting them to everyday sounds. These are known as 'assistive devices' and fall into four main categories.

1. TV aids and communicators – to enable an individual to turn up the volume of the TV or radio without disturbing other viewers or listeners. These can also be used by people talking with severely hearing impaired individuals and should be available in all clinics and wards, as well as to community-based staff to enable initial communication before appropriate referral.
2. Telephone aids – warning lights and/or extension bells to let people know when a telephone is ringing and devices that increase the volume of an incoming voice. Also faxes, and text telephones, such as Minicom, which allow two people who both have the machines to send a written message down the line.
3. Doorbell aids – flashing lights or additional bell units to let people know about callers at the door. This will be increasingly important with the expansion of community-based care.
4. Alarm aids – to enable an individual to be alerted to various types of alarms from clocks to smoke detectors. These use both flashing lights and vibrating units to alert people.

A few aids are available to individuals on permanent loan from social services, but this depends on the policy of the local department. Some local authorities may help with installation and rental costs under Section 2 of the Chronically Sick and Disabled Persons Act 1970. British Telecom also offer some services at reduced or no cost to customers with hearing impairment. Two schemes which help with running costs are 'Textphones for the Deaf' and 'Text Users Help Scheme' (details in Useful addresses). A wide range of devices is on display at the Royal National Institute for the Deaf (see Useful addresses). Close liaison with the medical social worker will ensure that patients have access to help to which they are entitled (see Chapter 12).

SUMMARY

The needs of the older population as they relate to audiology and hearing therapy services are simple. Older adults need to be able to communicate effectively so that they can function independently and live satisfying lives. Audiologists and hearing therapists can help them realize these goals by emphasizing and demonstrating interventions that are designed to achieve these ends.

REFERENCES

Alpiner, J.G. and McCarthy, P.A. (1993) *Rehabilitative Audiology for Children and Adults*, 2nd edn, Williams and Wilkins, Baltimore.

Bess, F., Lichtenstein, M. and Logan, S. (1991) Making hearing impairment functionally relevant: linkages with hearing disability and handicap. *Acta Otolaryngol (Stockh)* Suppl. **476**, 226–31.

HMSO (1994) *Direct Referral Systems for Hearing Aid Provision*, University of Manchester, Manchester.

Mulrow, C., Aguilar, C., Endicott, J. *et al.* (1990) Association between hearing impairment and the quality of the life of elderly individuals. *Journal of the American Geriatric Society*, **38**, 48–50.

Uhlmann, R., Larson, E., Rees, T., Koepsell, T. and Dukert, L. (1989) Relationship of hearing impairment to dementia and cognitive dysfunction in older adults. *Journal of the American Medical Association*, **261**, 1916–19.

Weinstein, B. and Amsell, L. (1986) Hearing loss and senile dementia in the institutionalised elderly. *Clinical Gerontology*, **4**, 3–15.

FURTHER READING

Ballantyne, J. (1977) *Deafness*, Churchill Livingstone, Edinburgh.

Bath and West Community NHS Trust (1993) *Hearing Therapy Service*, leaflet.

Cleggs, J., May, J., Pawluk, S. and Thurman, S. (undated) *Missing Out*, Brooklyn Press, Nottingham.

USEFUL ADDRESSES

RNID
105, Gower Street
London WC1E 6AH

Telephones for the Deaf
Royal National Institute for the Deaf
105, Gower Street
London WC1E 6AH

Text Users Rebate Scheme
Typetalk, National Telephone Relay Service
John Wood House
Glacier Building
Harrington Road
Brunswick Business Park
Liverpool L3 4DS

The role of the GP in primary care-led rehabilitation of older people

16

Chris Drinkwater

INTRODUCTION

The *Priorities and Planning Guidance* for the NHS 1996/97 (NHS Executive, 1995) identifies six medium-term priorities, of which two will have a significant impact on the rehabilitation of older people.

1. Work towards the development of a primary care-led NHS, in which decisions about the purchasing and provision of healthcare are taken as close to patients as possible.
2. Ensure in collaboration with local authorities and other organizations that integrated services are in place to meet needs for continuing healthcare and to allow elderly, disabled or vulnerable people to be supported in the community.

This is very much a changing NHS, in which GPs and primary health-care teams are being given a wider scope of influencing in the purchasing and provision of healthcare, within agreed priorities. At the same time there is also an expectation that the amount of institutional care, particularly long-stay NHS care, will decline and the resources released will be able to fund more flexible and appropriate care for patients within their local community. Inevitably this process, given the demographic trends which show increasing numbers of over 85s in the population, will mean that GPs will be caring for increasing numbers of patients who have higher levels of dependency. They are also going to have to address the problem of delivering comprehensive, integrated and cost-effective services to a group of people who often have multiple needs and require complex care packages.

This is a much more influential role than in the past. Historically general practice has functioned as a demand-led service, rather than a proactive, planned and managed service. This was recognized by a payment structure whereby GPs were (and still are) reimbursed additional capitation fees for patients over 65 and over 75, on the basis that this group make additional demands on workload. Although higher levels of demand were recognized, there was very little evaluation of need or targeting of those with highest levels of need. This led to a spate of publications in the 1960s and 1970s that identified high levels of unmet need in older patients registered with GPs. The response to this by a number of enthusiasts was the introduction of a variety of screening procedures to try to identify unmet need in older patients. This approach was finally formalized in the new General Practitioner Contract of 1989 which contained the requirement that all patients over 75 were to be offered an annual assessment to include mobility, special senses, continence and mental state. How this was to be done, who should do it, and what action was to be taken was left to the interpretation of individual practices. Anecdotal evidence suggests that a wide variety of approaches are being used and more formal research-based evidence suggests that if it is done properly, using validated instruments, it is very time consuming and not particularly cost effective in terms of the number of cases identified that need active intervention. The reasons for this latter finding are that a large number of people over 75 are active, fit and healthy. The group requiring intervention are very much a minority and they are often already known to their GP. The issue that now seems to be emerging is that need is identified, but is then unmet, for a combination of reasons, which include:

- lack of information about available services
- lack of understanding about the skills and competencies of other professionals, i.e. what have physiotherapy, occupational therapy and speech therapy got to offer? (see Chapters 9, 13 and 14).
- lack or shortage of appropriate services with consequent long waiting lists;
- inappropriate prosthetic response to need, for example provision of a walking frame for poor mobility, without proper assessment of whether mobility could be improved by a therapeutic intervention, such as altering or prescribing medication or referring for physiotherapy assessment.

A strong argument can be made that this situation will only change if and when primary healthcare teams begin to work more closely with all of the professions involved in the rehabilitation of older people. Joint working results in increased trust and understanding of the skills of other professions which should result in the more appropriate use and development of services. There is some evidence that this is already beginning to happen, particularly in fund holding practices which are in some cases beginning directly to commission physiotherapy, speech, chiropody and occupational therapy services.

WHY PRIMARY CARE-LED REHABILITATION?

Before considering how services might best be delivered in primary care, it is worth exploring whether this is a change for change sake, a change in order to control expensive secondary care costs or whether it might have definite benefits for patients. The strengths of primary care in respect of the care and rehabilitation of older people are as follows.

- There is a registered list of patients, which means that the size of the population can be identified and the likely level of need predicted.
- There is an easily accessible service, with responsibility 24 hours a day, 365 days of the year.
- There is continuity of care, often over many years. This results in high levels of trust and confidence, an important motivator in rehabilitation.
- There is an understanding and knowledge of patient and family dynamics and relationships. Problems in this area are often a cause of re-admission following rehabilitation in hospital.
- There is an ability to balance therapeutic optimism and realistic pessimism. The common caricature is the GP who is perceived to blame all problems on old age. This conveniently ignores the fact that growing old is often about coming to terms with functional disabilities for which there is no magical solution and that intervention can sometimes be misguided and harmful.
- There is greater sensitivity to patient autonomy, if only because the patient is within the familiar environment of their home or local practice, rather than in an alien hospital bed or clinic.
- There is core knowledge and skills within the team about the medical, nursing and preventive care of older people in the community.

These are all potential strengths and the fact that these strengths are not used or developed is also the greatest weakness of primary care-led rehabilitation of older people. Other weaknesses include:

- competing demands on time from other areas of work;
- lack of resources of accommodation and finance to deliver enhanced community-based services;
- a broader resource issue of dis-economies of scale: delivering services in patients' homes and in GPs' surgeries may be more expensive than delivering services from a central site;
- increasing pressure from ever-earlier hospital discharge, which may overload the system and result in breakdown (see Chapter 1);
- lack of appropriate knowledge and skills within the practice team about care of the elderly and more particularly about rehabilitation;
- undergraduate and postgraduate training for GPs in these areas is often very limited;

- poor links with social services, although this seems to have improved in some areas since the advent of Care in the Community;
- conflicts around professional power and autonomy which result in referrals for treatment rather than assessment by an autonomous colleague;
- wide variation between practices in the type of service that they offer.

This last point is illustrated by the fact that the balance sheet of strengths and weaknesses varies from practice to practice. The opportunities, however, are enormous. In many ways it is much easier to develop a new service than it is to change an existing hospital-based service, which is wedded to traditional patterns of delivery and where the overriding imperative is usually to try to get the patient out of hospital as quickly as possible.

WHAT SORT OF SERVICE SHOULD GPs BE DEVELOPING?

The best way of addressing this is to take a systems approach and to look at the critical transitions as patients move through the system. Falls in older people can be used as an example, by exploring four critical transition points.

1. Can falls be prevented or their effects ameliorated, thus avoiding entry into care?
2. If entry into care is required, can the patient be provided with a rapid and skilled assessment that results in an effective care plan?
3. Are appropriate arrangements in place to ensure effective discharge procedures from care?
4. What services need to be in place to maintain function and to prevent re-entry to care?

PREVENTION

Falls have a number of causes which may include uncoordination and poor mobility, cardiovascular and stroke disease, side-effects of medication, failing eyesight and dangers in the home such as frayed or loose carpets and poor lighting. All of these are to an extent preventable and there is increasing evidence of the effectiveness of prevention.

- Strength, stamina, skill and neuromuscular co-ordination may be improved by programmes of fitness training, thus decreasing the likelihood of falls.
- Increasing levels of physical activity can also help to prevent cardiovascular disease and stroke.

- Poor eyesight can be improved by assessment and provision of appropriate spectacles or by cataract operations.
- Safety in the home can be improved by the provision of advice, information and help.
- Assessment can be made and appropriate aids provided such as walking sticks and walking frames.
- Review can be carried out and, where appropriate, medication can be altered.

Prevention of the sequelae of falls

Maintaining strong bones, which are less likely to fracture, and being able to get up or to call for assistance after a fall are all ways of reducing the consequences of falls and provide opportunities for prevention. Bone density improves with physical activity and increased use of hormone replacement therapy also has a part to play. Those at risk of falls may be able to be taught how to rise from the ground or carers can be shown how to cope. This will improve confidence and prevent panic when a fall occurs. Frequent fallers and those who live alone may benefit from the provision of personal alarm systems or telephones within reach of the floor.

This brief exploration of the opportunities to prevent falls and their sequelae can be used to identify a number of professionals who have appropriate skills and might be involved in this area of work.

- Health visitors with health-promotion skills or Look after Yourself training might focus on strategies for increasing physical activity.
- Physiotherapists could also be involved in assessment procedures focused on increasing levels of physical activity as well as having a part to play in the provision of appropriate walking aids and in teaching people how to rise from the ground after a fall.
- Opticians need to be involved in assessment and provision of appropriate spectacles.
- Occupational therapists could be involved in assessing risk and providing advice about the prevention of accidents in the home.
- Pharmacists could be involved in review of medication.
- Social workers need to be involved in assessment for and provision of personal alarms and telephones.

The main barriers to getting these groups together to deliver a preventive service are the limited incentives to practise prevention and the need to find someone to take responsibility for co-ordinating and delivering the service.

NEED FOR ASSESSMENT AND CARE

In the systems model, if prevention has failed and the patient now needs care, the next critical point is access to appropriate care. Following a fall, access to services is most commonly through two different pathways: through a GP practice or the accident and emergency (A&E) department of a hospital.

GP assessment may result in referral to secondary care if there are broken bones or the patient has had a stroke. Often, however, the patient is simply stiff, sore and frightened. This may result in a disabling loss of mobility, which results in an immediate need for home care and/or district nursing support. Early assessment by a physiotherapist may also be required, in order to prevent the vicious cycle of loss of confidence resulting in poor gait and/or immobility which will inevitably increase the risk of further falls.

Depending on circumstances, attendance at an A&E department will either result in admission to hospital or assessment, treatment and return home. The general practice perception of this process is that often insufficient account is taken of social and family circumstances and that before sending a patient who lives alone home with a plaster on their arm, a care plan which may involve social services is likely to be required. Occupational therapists working in conjunction with A&E departments are able to offer such a service, preventing the need for admission.

This point in the system produces another list of professionals:

- The GP or A&E doctor with responsibility for medical assessment;
- The district nurse, providing skilled nursing care at home;
- The physiotherapist, providing early assessment and intervention to restore mobility and increase self confidence;
- The social worker, providing a social care assessment with access where necessary to skilled home care support;
- The occupational therapist, assessing the need for early home adaptations.

All of these groups have skills and expertise to offer, but if the patient is to receive an appropriate and effective package of care, it is essential that this care is co-ordinated and that the professionals involved communicate with one another and work together as a team.

DISCHARGE FROM HOSPITAL

If the patient has now been admitted to hospital, the next critical point is discharge home. This is happening at ever earlier points which inevitably reduces the margin of error, making it even more important to get the care plan right and in place before the patient goes home. Failure at this point usually results in rapid re-admission or inappropriate placement in residential or nursing care. One of the most common and often overlooked reasons for failure is a misperception of the difference between primary and secondary care. The patient in the hospital bed has been rehabilitated, is desperately keen to go home and puts on a wonderful performance. The carer at home is anxious, uncertain and frequently over-caring and the GP and the district nurse are concerned about carers' ability to cope. The pre-discharge home assessment visit goes some way to addressing this issue, but too often the focus is on functional and instrumental issues rather than on patient/carer psychology and psychodynamics. Unless these issues are acknowledged and addressed, if necessary by providing additional support, then the result is usually failure.

Another general issue in this area is the cost of complex home-based care packages and early discharge packages when a large amount of health and social care is still required. These packages are often more expensive than institutional care and increasingly social service departments are putting a ceiling on costs and insisting on a review when the cost of domiciliary care exceeds the cost of nursing home care. It is equally likely that fund holders, particularly the total fund-holding pilots, will wish to impose limits on domiciliary medical care packages where these are more expensive than institutional care.

Other issues that are important for good discharge practice include:

- good rapid communication systems between secondary and primary care, which should include information about what the patient and their carer have been told;
- rapid provision of aids and appliances and, if more complex household adaptations are required (provision of a stairlift, for example), an agreed plan and time scale for doing this;
- agreement on a continuing home-based rehabilitation package and clear identification of the person providing the package;
- good communication between providers of health and social care, either through a key worker or a care manager;
- an agreed mechanism for reviewing the care package after a certain time or in response to changing needs.

Clearly a number of different professionals need to be involved in the process but the key issues concern good communication between patients and carers and between members of the team. To some extent this is about ensuring that good systems are in place and that they are regularly reviewed, but the more important issue is often about attitudes and values as barriers to better inter-professional working. In the long term, the best way of tackling this is through inter-professional education.

MAINTENANCE OF FUNCTION

The final part of the system is about maintaining the gains achieved through rehabilitation. From a primary care perspective this is often an area that is overlooked. The common pattern is rehabilitation followed by a gradual decline in function which at some stage triggers the need for a further intensive episode of rehabilitation. If anything this is becoming more of a problem, with targeted and costed brief interventions becoming the purchasing norm. This makes it very difficult to develop a service that contains a costing for a regular review or support visit, which is focused on educational reinforcement of patient and carer and maintenance of morale. The fact that chronic visiting of house-bound patients remains a part of primary care attests to the value that patients and their carers place on this sort of service, despite the fact that it is often resented by GPs, who see it as social visiting where nothing medically useful takes place.

The other important area where maintenance of function is a major problem is nursing home care. There are three reasons for this. First, placement in a nursing home is often seen as an end point, providing professionals with an opportunity to withdraw and concentrate on the next case. Second, although regular re-assessment should be part of all nursing home packages of care, this is usually the area that is abandoned if pressure in other parts of the system, such as discharge arrangements, becomes overwhelming. Third, there is difficulty of access by nursing homes and their residents to therapy services. The main issue concerns charging structures and the common practice of listing these services as an addition to nursing home care, with the result that costs are passed on to the patient or their relatives.

Problems in this area are likely to increase as a consequence of new arrangements for continuing care which will result in greater numbers of high-dependency patients being placed in nursing homes. Unless this issue of access to therapy services is resolved, it is likely to have a detrimental effect on the quality of life of patients in nursing homes.

A COMMUNITY REHABILITATION SERVICE

The previous sections of this chapter have identified the need for a community rehabilitation service. This section will explore how such a service might be provided and funded. At present a number of fund-holding, multi-fund and total fund-holding practices are either buying in services from Community Trusts or developing their own services. The scope of these developments are very variable and where practices are employing their own therapy staff this raises all sorts of issues for practices about ensuring the competence of people they employ, providing them with appropriate equipment, training and professional development and support, not to mention annual leave and sickness cover.

The other possible model is to develop a community team with responsibility for a particular locality or grouping of practices. We already have community mental health teams, so why not community care of the elderly teams? These would be multidisciplinary teams with a full range of professionals: nursing, geriatrician, physiotherapy, occupational therapy, speech therapy, chiropody and social services. Other possible additions to this team could include general practice input to build bridges with the practices and psychology input to provide support around the behavioural and motivational issues that can occur when providing community care to dependent and disabled people.

The advantage of such a team is that it would begin to break down inter-professional barriers and would ensure better communication between the different professionals who might be involved in the delivery of a complex care package. This approach would also simplify and improve multidisciplinary assessment as well as improving access to a range of therapists by primary care teams. In the longer term this sort of team could also begin to enhance knowledge and skills in primary care teams, and residential and nursing homes through educational and audit approaches. Because of a locality approach there would also be opportunities for developing links with voluntary sector services and perhaps even for taking on some of the issues around health promotion and illness prevention.

SUMMARY

The number of older people in the community together with their complex problems is increasing. More of these people live alone and informal care is more problematic, because the main carer is often elderly, and social expectations and traditions around family support are changing. Against this background, national policy for both health and social services has been to move away from institutional care to integrated services, which allow vulnerable older people to be supported in the community. The other main policy change has been to give GPs greater responsibility for the purchasing of health care.

These changes leave the GP in a unique position to co-ordinate a team of autonomous professionals for expert assessment with a view to providing appropriate care, preventing further problems, promoting health and maximizing independence. The 'faller' is used as a case example. A Community Care of the Elderly Team is proposed as a possible model for providing a cost-effective locally based service.

REFERENCE

NHS Executive (1995) *Priorities and Planning Guidance for the NHS: 1995/96*, EL(95)68, Department of Health, Leeds.

Overview and future of rehabilitation of older people

17

Amanda J. Squires

BACKGROUND

The history of rehabilitation of older people in the UK has evolved from the care of the poor by religious institutions in the Medieval era, and Poor Law provision in the Middle Ages. Demographic changes in the latter half of the 20th century have resulted in not only escalating numbers of older people, both indigenous and of ethnic minorities, but also their attendant health and social problems, their need for functional ability to remain independent, their rising expectations and the shortage of both formal and informal carers to meet these needs.

REFORM OF HEALTH AND SOCIAL CARE

Like many national health systems, the NHS responded to the mismatch between supply and demand by instituting reform. It was hoped that the resulting market culture would improve efficiency and at the same time raise standards. The reforms have provided opportunities for new ways of working, and have also identified the need for additional skills – both clinical and commercial. Initially, rehabilitation will remain hospital based, but as the re-allocation of resources promotes change, and community teams develop, rehabilitation services will need to respond. At the time of writing, such changes are in the early stages of development and traditional services are described, with a vision of what the future might entail.

HEALTHCARE FOR OLDER PEOPLE

The principles of healthcare for older people are based on the existence of their good health, the possibility of multiple pathology, the need for accurate diagnosis, the need for comprehensive functional assessment, the need for effective and timely team work by specialists to implement care plans at a pace compatible with the capacity of the older person to respond and the involvement of older people and their carers in health promotion.

ETHICAL CONSIDERATIONS

Traditional values within health and social care are being challenged by social changes. Practitioners already working autonomously, as a result of the unique multipathology and multidimensional social influences of older people, will increasingly have to face ethical questions about their decisions. Professional codes of ethics provide guidelines for such decision making, and the issues – seldom taught in basic training – will need to be considered and debated by teams of practitioners.

TEAM WORK

As the traditional membership of rehabilitation teams changes as a result of reform, and especially through new providers entering the market, cohesiveness will be even more important, to provide benefit for all stakeholders. Users should be unaware of 'seams' between providers or agencies in the packages of care they receive. The formation, development and outcome of teams will no longer be optional, but will need planning and evaluation. This must build on classic theories, making them relevant by providing practical tips for success such as clear objectives, ongoing monitoring of progress, identification of needed skills, robust membership selection processes, training and leadership for successful and enjoyable work.

ASSESSMENT, GOALS AND OUTCOMES

Multidisciplinary assessment is the key to the formulation of shared goals and consistent treatment plans acceptable to the older person, informal and formal carers. The danger of gaps and duplications occurring when a number of people are involved can be avoided by use of key workers and accurate and timely communication. The optimal outcome of the process will be increasingly sought by all stakeholders, but is disconcertingly complex and must be appropriate to the work of all members of the team.

MENTAL HEALTH

Mental health problems may be identified by any member of the team and all should be aware of the common issues that surround the mental well being of older people. Physical ability and mental health are interlinked and assessment findings must be used to adjust treatment plans, and their method of implementation. The consequences of the effect of the patient's illness on carers should also be included in the assessment and support for their input facilitated wherever possible.

COMMUNICATION AND SPEECH AND LANGUAGE THERAPY

Communication is essential, both for team co-ordination and in relation to users, for successful care plan implementation. The everyday function of communication is the result of complex and largely unconscious processes. During normal ageing, only some of these processes are affected, and to widely varying degrees. These include such things as speed of processing information and biological changes affecting voice production. Speech and language therapists can help in the differential diagnosis and treatment of such clinical problems and can also give team members and carers some insight into how their own communication style can be enhanced to improve interaction. Feeding and swallowing are an additional problem which appropriate management can improve, thus increasing well being and reducing the anxiety of both formal and informal carers, who may be responsible for providing food and fluids.

NURSING

The nurse has a key role in rehabilitation, being able to contribute a unique view to the assessment, as well as consistent implementation of appropriate parts of the plan. Basic nursing skills applied 'to' the patient are rapidly becoming more aimed at 'enhancing' the patient's functional ability. This is exemplified in the move from task to team and currently to primary methods of organization.

FEET, FOOT CARE, FOOTWEAR AND CHIROPODY

Assessment is not complete unless the feet and footwear are included. Mobility is the key to independence and relies on comfortable feet and safe footwear. Older people bring with them a lifetime of trauma to their feet, and may also have symptoms of other disorders such as diabetes and rheumatoid arthritis. Identification of need may be for basic self care or professional intervention by a chiropodist. Carers should be encouraged to continue basic hygiene care of the feet, perhaps in conjunction with chiropody. Adequate footwear should be available to complement foot care and enhance safe mobility. Retail and bespoke footwear address each end of the range of foot problems, but seldom the centre. A cost-effective scheme is described that enables timely provision of safe footwear following a comprehensive assessment.

SOCIAL CARE

Social work is carried out within considerable legal constraints developed to protect vulnerable individuals. This background may be at odds with those of other team members, especially at the community/hospital inter-face either at admission or at discharge. The reform of social care has empowered social services to act as both purchaser and provider of care for those in need, but much is means tested with its attendant conse-quences. The focus is now on the development of packages of care to enable older people to live at home where possible and this is in line with the views of health service colleagues. The full service cost has yet to be realized, both in equipment and in human resources.

PHYSIOTHERAPY

The skill of the physiotherapist with older people is the ability to assess and interpret the problems of movement caused by multiple factors, and to provide appropriate intervention for functional gain in line with the team plan. The training of other healthcare workers to encourage appro-priate functional activity within their programmes will increase in line with community-based care and the drive for efficiency. The move to pri-mary care provides opportunities for earlier intervention to promote health and prevent disability, and is reliant on an understanding by team members already in contact with the potential patient to make timely and appropriate referral.

OCCUPATIONAL THERAPY

Occupational therapists work either for the NHS or for local authorities. NHS services focus on assessment and programmes to meet the personal, domestic, social, psychological and physical needs of those undergoing rehabilitation. Local authority services work to statutory and local require-ments dealing witih clients with disabilities needing minor and major home adaptations, the needs of their carers, and the needs of the wider disabled population, ensuring physical access to community facilities.

OTHER KEY SERVICES

The core services for rehabilitation of the older patient are complemented by a number of others, in particular:

- *Nutrition and dietetics*, to aid recovery, maintain health and adapt to changed dietary intake, such as from swallowing difficulties following stroke;

- *Dentistry*, for social as well as nutritional benefit, and to promote and maintain health;
- *Pharmacy*, for appropriate prescription advice and awareness of side-effects and prescription compliance. Older people are likely to have complex pharmacy intake. Advice to team members who have little experience of this subject may be helpful, especially as the results of medication may be best determined by changes in functional ability;
- *Continence problems*, frequently the cause of admission to institutional care, and a barrier to discharge, and may be the result of factors potentially influenced by other team members, e.g. diet, medication, mobility and home adaptations. Accurate diagnosis, treatment and re-assessment are essential, as is feedback from team members on progress.
- *Hearing services*, essential for diagnosis, provision and maintenance of hearing aids when appropriate and rehabilitation, to maximize hearing and facilitate wider rehabilitation and social integration;
- *Optical services*, frequently overlooked by older people and their formal and informal carers. They are essential for both diagnosis and the provision and maintenance of aids, most commonly spectacles, to maximize sight to facilitate wider rehabilitation and safety.

GENERAL PRACTITIONERS

Primary care is beginning to address the increasing numbers of older people, who with their elderly carers will take part in rehabilitation programmes in the community. GPs will be in a unique position to co-ordinate a team of autonomous professionals in prevention, diagnosis, assessment and care planning. For such a multidisciplinary approach in a complex environment to be successful from the viewpoint of all stakeholders, knowledge of and respect for the work of colleagues will be essential.

CONCLUSION AND RECOMMENDATIONS

What is clear from the contributions to this book is that all the key services involved are jointly addressing the functional problems of older people in a variety of ways, and often against social and professional prejudice. For each of these services, assessment, goal setting and treatment planning in conjunction with the older person, formal and informal carers is essential. The agreed plan of treatment must be personalized, implemented consistently and regularly reviewed. The contributors to an older person's care plan need to work in a co-ordinated way to achieve effectiveness, efficiency and value for the older person and their carers. Each service has its outcome measures, but for the patient, only their view of the expected outcome is important, and evaluation of a quality service should be from that perspective. Teams will therefore need to work towards shared, patient-centred goals and their measures of successful achievement.

As community-based rehabilitation of older people and the market approach to healthcare delivery develops, the co-ordination of services will become even more important and the GP, community nurse and care manager will play pivotal roles. All those involved will need to have an understanding of the contributions available, criteria for referral and the ensuing process, so as to be able to make appropriate referrals, and to ensure that consistent information is presented to the potential user. The sharing of appropriate skills will enable a more cost-effective approach to be taken by qualified staff, so long as access to expert help is available. More use will need to be made of unqualified, but trained, assistants to carry out appropriate routine work under supervision. A generic approach will enable implementation of such care, delegated by a number of disciplines. This has a number of problems, such as accountability, supervision and training which need to be overcome for success. Informal carers will also have an expanding role, and their training and support will become more important as the numbers and felt needs of older people increase.

Providers, both traditional and non-traditional, will be commissioned for variable periods and will need to integrate, and feel welcome, at the start of the contract period. Accurate documentation is essential and will be needed to ensure that effective handover between departing and arriving providers is adequate.

The Health Service Ombudsman regularly reports that complaints about the service are mainly about lack of, or inconsistency of, information, and about staff attitudes. Addressing this in community-based care will set even bigger challenges. An undertaking of the work of the key disciplines involved will address the former, and the 'good practice' examples within this book encouraging effectiveness, efficiency and enthusiasm should address the latter.

Successful rehabilitation of the older person will be based on a timely and appropriate response to the needs of the older person and their carers.

Index

Page numbers appearing in **bold** refer to figures and page numbers appearing in *italic* refer to tables.